In Gratitude

I am in deep gratitude to the following individuals who are courageous enough to publicly question the safety and effectiveness of vaccines. This list includes doctors, research scientists, politicians, parents and concerned citizens who risk their reputations and livelihoods to tell the truth.

Andrew Wakefield MD, Brian Hooker Ph.D., Tony Bark MD
Polly Tommy, Robert Sears MD, Anita Bratt ND
Michael Leitner, James Lyons-Weiler Ph.D., Leon Chaitow
Suzanne Humphries MD, Roman Bystrianyk, Paul Thomas MD
Neil Z. Miller, Gary Goldman Ph.D., Robert F. Kennedy Jr.
Robert De Niro, Sherri J. Tenpenny MD, Walene James
Tetyana Obukhanych Ph.D., Brett Wilcox, Lauren Feder MD
David Kirby, Dan Olmsted, Mark Blaxill, Mary Holland JD
Kent Heckenlively, Judy Mikovits Ph.D., Alan Cassels
Marcia Angell MD, David Lewis Ph.D., Linda Keller, Dan Burton
Steven Druker, Kevin Barry, Sharyl Attkisson, Heather Fraser
Andrew Moulden MD Ph.D., Vernon Coleman MD, Anne Dachel
Jenny McCarthy, Edda West, Rita Hoffman, Nelle Maxey
Claudina Michal-Teitelbaum MD, Richard Moskowitz MD
Larry Palevksy MD, Todd M. Elsner DC, Philip F. Incao MD
Barbara Loe Fisher, Ralph Campbell MD, Gregory Polland MD
Russell Blaylock MD, Judy Converse MPH, Elliott Freed
Peter Doshi Ph.D., Michael Crichton MD, Robert Mendelsohn MD
Larry Solomon, Meryl Nass MD, Del Bigtree, Joel Lord
Lorna Hancock, Aviva Jill Romm, Laura Hayes, Tim Sullivan
Chris Shaw Ph.D., Jayne Donegan MD, and many others

During times of universal deceit,
telling the truth becomes a revolutionary act.

~ George Orwell, 1984

There is no greater power than a community
discovering what it cares about.

~ Margaret J. Wheatley

Dedication

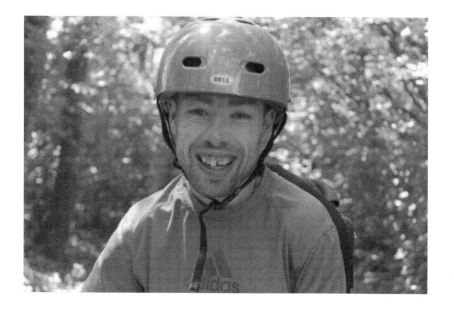

In memory of
Joshua Anthony Kuntz
July 25, 1984 – February 16, 2017

A beautiful son.
An amazing teacher.
Sacrificed for 'the greater good'.

Most institutions demand unqualified faith;
but the institution of science makes skepticism
a virtue.

~ Robert King Merton

Table of Contents

The secret of freedom lies in educating people,
whereas the secret of tyranny is in keeping them ignorant.

~ Robespierre

WARNING:

This book may require thinking for yourself.

Ask your Doctor if thinking for yourself
is right for you.

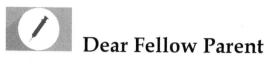 Dear Fellow Parent

Thank you for your courage and curiosity in considering the information contained in this book. Your willingness to open yourself to this information is a gift to your family. I have a core belief that everyone does the best they can with what they know. The challenge of life is that we are often required to make decisions without adequate information.

You might ask what my intention is in writing this book. The answer is – I want you to be as informed as possible about the medical practice of vaccination. I also want to defend your right to informed consent.

I appreciate there may be some hesitation in considering this information. We've been dare I say, indoctrinated to believe that vaccines are safe and effective; that the benefits outweigh the risks; that we have a social responsibility to vaccinate; and that without vaccines our children's lives would be at risk.

Our need to protect our children from harm makes it exceedingly challenging to consider ideas we have been told repeatedly will cause significant injury or even the death of our children.

I once thought as you do. I accepted without question the messages from conventional medical providers, the vaccine industry, politicians and the mainstream media. I trusted these individuals and organizations when they said vaccines are safe and effective and essential to ensuring the health and safety of our children.

Dare to Question

I thought this until my son Josh was permanently harmed by the DPT vaccine at five months of age. The vaccine caused significant neurological injury that Josh never recovered from. Josh lived with an uncontrolled seizure disorder and required 24-hour care for his entire life. My son never got to experience a full and healthy life.

The DPT vaccine changed both his life and mine in ways I never imagined when we consented to that first vaccination. Josh passed away in February 2017 from his vaccine related injuries. As a result of the significant neurological injuries caused by the DPT vaccine, the United States and Canadian governments eventually replaced the vaccine with the DtaP acellular pertussis vaccine, thought to be less harmful. Their action, however, was too late for my son and many others.

We all want our children to be happy, healthy and successful. After years of research I've come to the conclusion that our children's health is not dependent on injecting them with a complex mixture of biological and neurotoxic substances to artificially stimulate their immune system.

Rather, our children's health is dependent on our willingness to take responsibility for our health and that of our children, the courage to ask questions, and our ability to gather sufficient information to make well-informed decisions.

Global Effort to Eliminate Informed Consent

The fact is there is a well-organized, industry-funded effort to eliminate your right to medical decision-making and self-determination with regard to the vaccination of your children. Efforts are underway in countries around the world to remove free will and impose vaccinations on you and your children. The *Pediatric Alliance of Ontario* has openly declared this is one of their goals for 2017/18.

California, Australia, France and Italy have all recently enacted legislation to make the state the primary vaccine decision-maker and deprive parents of their right and responsibility to decide what medical interventions they will subject their children to.

Civil liberties . . . we shall enjoy them
only so long as we value them enough to preserve them.

~ George W. Brown

If you believe vaccines really are as safe and effective as claimed, you may not have any concern with surrendering your right to medical decision-making. But if vaccines are not nearly as safe, effective or necessary, and not as evidence-based as claimed, then you may want to preserve your right to medical decision-making for yourself and your children.

Unlike the medical industry, the media and our politicians, I have no financial interest in what you decide. I only want what is best for you and your family. I only wish that your family not experience what my family experienced.

As you read through this material I anticipate you will discover there is much about vaccines and the vaccine industry you didn't know or were never told. This experience is not uncommon. Open and honest discussion about vaccine safety, effectiveness and necessity is actively discouraged. The media censors any public criticism, concern, or debate about vaccine safety and effectiveness.

But what if what we've been told isn't true? What if the science doesn't support mass universal vaccination? What if the medical community is not in unanimous agreement about the safety, effectiveness and need for vaccinations? What if the efforts to impose mandatory vaccination are motivated by financial interests rather than improved health?

Dare to Question

What if the growing epidemic of chronic illness, immune and neurological injury, and sudden infant death are a result of the massive increase in the number of vaccines our children are exposed to? What if vaccinated children are not healthier than unvaccinated children?

The decision of whether or not to vaccinate is the most important decision you will make as a parent.

Are you prepared? Do you have enough information? Do you have solid, verifiable evidence to be confident in your decision? The challenge of vaccination is that this decision cannot be undone.

As a young parent I didn't question the vaccine decision. I didn't educate myself about this medical practice. I simply went along and did what I was told was expected of me. I didn't take responsibility for the decision to vaccinate my son.

Regretfully, I came to the information in this book too late for my son and my family. I want better for you and your family. I want you to be informed, aware, and a parent who consciously chooses what is in your children's best interest.

But first you must 'dare to question' everything you've been told about the practice of artificial immune stimulation.

Sincerely,

Ted Kuntz, father of Joshua

> *When I tell the truth it is not for the sake of*
> *convincing those who do not know it,*
> *but for the sake of defending those that do.*
>
> ~ William Blake

In Recognition of Parents

Passionate amateurs are motivated by necessity
and inspired by love.
Someone or something they care about is vulnerable,
under siege or in trouble,
and they have no choice but to respond.

Passionate amateurs don't quit. They can't quit.
They are prepared to pour their life's energy
into resolving a challenge.
Their commitment is freely given.

They are on the front lines, spotting and dealing
with injustice years and sometimes decades
before the issue seeps into the consciousness
of organizations and institutions.
They experience or witness the barriers and
system failures first-hand.

They know that slow, incremental change isn't good enough
for the people, places and creatures they love.

~ Al Etmanski
Author of *Impact*

I never imagined myself in this position,
least so in the very beginning
of my Ph.D. research training in immunology.
In fact, at that time, I was very enthusiastic
about the concept of vaccination,
just like any typical immunologist.

However, after years of doing research in immunology,
observing scientific activities of my superiors,
and analyzing vaccine issues,
I realized that vaccination is
one of the most deceptive inventions
that science could ever convince the world to accept.

~ Dr. Tetyana Obukhanych, Ph. D.
Author of *Vaccine Illusion*

Making an Informed Choice

The vaccine paradigm is based upon an *assumption* that injecting a complex mixture of biological and neurotoxic substances will protect humans from infectious disease.

While there is evidence that some vaccines have been effective in the suppression of disease symptoms, the total impact of the artificial stimulation of the human immune system has not been adequately investigated and is not well understood or established.

The artificial immunization program was developed more than two hundred years ago when virtually nothing was known about the impact of injecting complex biochemical substances, foreign DNA, and toxins on organs, the neurological and immune systems, and at the cellular level.

Today, we have irrefutable evidence that the ingredients in vaccines can and do cause harm, even death. This is evidenced by the more than $3.7 billion in compensation paid to vaccine-injured individuals in the United States by the US National Vaccine Injury Compensation Program. [1] And we know this amount represents only a small fraction of the total number of vaccine injury victims who are rarely acknowledged, much less compensated.

As more evidence of vaccine injury is acknowledged, there is increasing consideration being given by parents and some medical professionals to modify the recommended CDC vaccine schedule. Is it reasonable to propose a modified or delayed vaccine schedule in response to vaccine injury? Or is it time to question the very basis of the artificial immune stimulation program?

This book is written by a parent and is for parents. I've spent more than thirty years reviewing the vaccine literature. *'Dare to Question'* offers an overview of the many questions and concerns related to the practice of artificial immune stimulation, more commonly referred to as vaccination.

This information is presented in response to the following questions:

> Vaccinations - Science or Religion?
> Am I the Only One?
> Is the Delivery System Safe?
> Is Vaccine Science Trustworthy?
> Is the Measles Crisis Real?
> Is Vaccine Policy Sound?
> Is the Claim of Safety Valid?
> Are Vaccines Effective?
> Is Vaccine History Accurate?
> Can Vaccine Oversight Be Trusted?
> Where Do We Go From Here?
> If Not Vaccines, Then What?
> Where Can I Get More Information?

The decision to vaccinate or not is one of the most important decisions a responsible parent is required to make. I offer the following information for your thoughtful consideration.

We know that parents who vaccinate their children sincerely believe they are protecting their child from harm. They believe vaccines will provide a type of health insurance, shielding their child from disease.

At Vaccine Choice Canada we think it is important that we push beyond using "belief" as the basis for the vaccine decision, and instead decide from a place of information based on quality scientific evidence.

~ Edda West, Co-founder
Vaccine Choice Canada

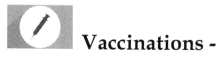

Vaccinations - Science or Religion?

We pride ourselves on being more intelligent, more conscious and more evolved than the human beings who came before us. We find it deplorable that previous generations believed in bloodletting, lobotomy, exorcism, forced sterilization, slavery, criminalization of homosexuals, and the divine right of Kings and Queens.

Have we fully evolved? Are there no other areas of blindness, dogma, false belief, or unsubstantiated claims of what everyone 'knows to be true'? What might we accept today as truth that a future generation will find incredulous and dismiss as the thinking of a primitive species?

One practice I propose future generations will undoubtedly question is our current preoccupation with injecting a mixture of viruses, chemical preservatives, animal products, heavy metals and neurotoxins into the human body, especially our infants and children. We refer to this practice as vaccination.

Many readers will scoff at this statement. They will treat any expression of concern about the safety and effectiveness of vaccinations as the ranting of a lunatic, Luddite, anti-science fool who ought to be immediately silenced and dismissed. Such is the power of the belief in the *'miracle of vaccinations'*.

The belief in vaccinations is so strong that even discussion of the issue is denied. Mainstream medicine aggressively suppresses any debate on the safety, effectiveness and necessity of vaccines.

Dare to Question

So convinced are we on the merits of vaccination that an active censorship exists to prevent giving voice to those who might entertain such 'false beliefs'.

"There is consensus in the medical community," we are told. *"All vaccines are safe and effective."* End of story. No further discussion or investigation is needed or desired. Allowing discussion and debate would give credibility where no credibility is due. This would be 'false balance'.

The typical messages that are routinely delivered by the pharmaceutical industry and mainstream media whenever questions of vaccine safety are raised are –

X   Vaccines are safe and effective.
X   Vaccine injury is one in a million.
X   The benefits of vaccination far outweigh the risks.
X   We have a social responsibility to vaccinate.
X   The science on vaccines is clear.
X   Vaccines do not cause autism.

Unfortunately none of these statements are scientific facts.

These statements are opinions and promotional statements.
They are propaganda masquerading as science.

Saying all vaccines are safe and effective is like saying all prescription drugs are safe and effective. The statement also implies that all vaccines are safe and effective for all people, which obviously isn't true given the US Vaccine Court has awarded more than 3.7 billion dollars in compensation for vaccine injury since 1989.

Anyone who states – *"the science regarding vaccinations is clear"* is not a scientist, nor being honest.

———

The undisputed facts are the following:

- There are no long-term clinical trials that prove vaccine safety.

- Most effectiveness trials are limited to the measurement of anti-bodies in the blood rather than producing verifiable evidence that the vaccine actually prevented the targeted disease.

- No safety trials exist that determine the safety of giving multiple vaccinations at once.

- No large safety trials using an unvaccinated population as the control group have proven that vaccines are safe and effective.

- The current vaccine schedule has never been tested for safety in the real world way in which the schedule is implemented.

- No clinical proof exists to support the claim that vaccines are responsible for the decline in mortality, let alone the claim of millions of lives saved.

- There are no clinical studies that show injecting mercury into humans is safe in any amount.

- The amount of aluminum used in vaccines regularly exceeds the maximum amount permitted by the FDA.

Unfortunately facts are not part of the discussion because there is no discussion. Vaccination is effectively a religion. Doctors and the pharmaceutical industry are the new high priests.

Dare to Question

It is blasphemy to question the edicts of the high priests. The punishment for questioning is being silenced, ostracized and banished.

Everyone must believe. Anyone who does not believe is deemed a threat to the community. Fear of damnation is used to coerce compliance with the prevailing dogma. Laws must be put in place to secure the compliance of those who do not believe.

Parents in California are no longer able to decide what is injected into their children without forfeiting their right to a public education. This means children in California do not belong to their parents. Children are the property of the State.

The strength of this dogma will be evident in the emotional response to this essay. Many will immediately dismiss what is presented here. The dismissal will not be based on verifiable scientific evidence. It will not be based on well-designed and critically evaluated clinical trials of safety and effectiveness. Rather the dismissal will be based on a *belief* of what everyone knows to be true. No evidence is required to confirm what everyone already knows to be true.

Then in some future time when a shift in consciousness occurs, the thought of injecting toxins into our infants and children will be viewed as highly irresponsible and relegated to the mysteries of a primitive species alongside bloodletting, the superiority of one race over another, and the belief that we are the centre of the universe.

The challenge of being asleep is that you don't know you are asleep until you wake up.

Just because you believe what you've been told,
doesn't make it true.

Am I The Only One?

We must leave room for doubt
or there is no progress and no learning.
There is no learning without having to pose a question,
and a question requires doubt.

~ Richard Feynman
Nobel Prize Winner 1965

Many Parents Question Vaccines

You might reasonably wonder if you are the only parent questioning vaccine safety and effectiveness. The mainstream media intentionally marginalizes people who question vaccine safety and effectiveness with labels like: *anti-vaccine, anti-vaxxer, anti-science, irresponsible, misguided, uninformed*, etc.

The fact is there are many parents who are questioning vaccine safety, effectiveness and necessity. The medical journal, *Pediatrics*, reports:

> *The number of pediatricians encountering parents who question vaccine safety, refuse one or more vaccines, or want to use an alternative vaccination schedule increased from just under* **75%** *in 2006 to* **87%** *by 2013.* [1]

The number of parents questioning the safety, effectiveness and necessity of vaccines is even higher today.

Is Questioning Vaccine Safety New?

Concern about vaccine safety and the loss of the right to informed consent and self-determination is not new.

In the 1800s, there was public criticism of the smallpox vaccine. People objected for the same reasons as they do today, on the basis of scientific, religious, political and health concerns.

In 1853 in Victorian England, *The Vaccination Act* introduced mandatory vaccination of infants. There was immediate resistance. Parents demanded the right to control their bodies and those of their children. Anti-mandatory vaccination organizations were formed to end forced vaccination.

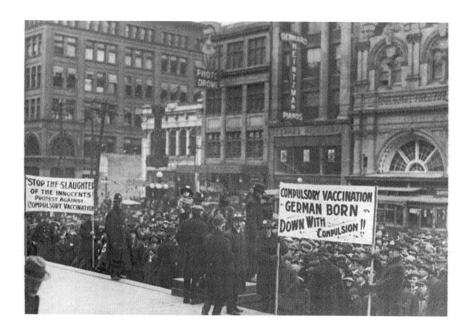

Protest Against Compulsory Vaccination - Toronto, Canada.
November 13, 1919

Its Not Just Parents Questioning Vaccines

And it's not just parents who are questioning the safety, effectiveness and necessity of vaccines. Other organizations and professional bodies are challenging the claims of the Centre for Disease Control and the pharmaceutical industry.

Public health officials and the medical profession have abrogated their professional, public, and human responsibility, by failing to honestly examine the iatrogenic harm caused by expansive, indiscriminate, and increasingly aggressive vaccination policies.

On a human level, the documented evidence shows a callous disregard for the plight of thousands of children who suffer irreversible harm, as if they were unavoidable "collateral damage".

Dare to Question

*The corrupting influence of the pharmaceutical industry on
medical research and its published literature, has derailed
the medical profession from its humanitarian mission
and its professional objectivity.* [2]

~ Alliance for Human Research Protection

Many physicians have come together to form *'Physicians for Informed Consent'*. Their vision is to - *"Live in a society free of mandatory vaccination laws."*

These physicians recognize that mandatory vaccination laws threaten our health, our rights and our liberty. *Physicians for Informed Consent* is a member of a coalition of more than 70 local, national and international organizations that recognize the importance of informed consent and are dedicated to protecting and preserving that right.

Physicians for Informed Consent is not ideologically pro-vaccine or anti-vaccine. Rather, they are pro-health, pro-ethics and pro-informed consent in vaccination, as in any other medical procedure.

*Informed consent involves the basic human right
to consent or refuse a medical treatment
or procedure, including vaccination.
The consent must be voluntary.*

*If a patient, or parent of a patient, is coerced or threatened
in any way into consenting for vaccination
(including statutory or government mandated exclusion from school),
then the "consent" obtained
is actually coerced consent, not informed consent.*

~ Physicians for Informed Consent

Why Isn't This Information Reported in the Media?

This is a good question. The short answer is – *'follow the money'*. The mainstream media rely on advertising revenues to stay in business. The pharmaceutical industry is one of the largest sources of advertising revenues today.

Robert F. Kennedy Jr. reported that in a non-election year in the United States, mainstream news programs receive 70% of their advertising revenues from the pharmaceutical industry. A top-level television executive admitted to Kennedy that he would dismiss any producer who aired a program that put their pharmaceutical advertising revenues at risk.

There is intense pressure exerted on media, including social media (Google, Facebook, Pinterest), to censor vaccine concern and criticism. Seth Berkley, director of GAVI, an international alliance of vaccine manufacturers has called for "anti-vaxxers" to be banned from all social media.

The vaccine industry hires 'internet trolls' who literally troll the Internet to mock and vilify anyone who expresses concern about vaccine safety, effectiveness or necessity. These industry trolls undermine our right to freedom of speech.

Vaccine Safety Science is Hazardous

Scientists examining vaccine safety report they are routinely attacked because of their efforts to investigate vaccine safety. These authors state that, rather than the science being critiqued, they are being attacked personally. This sends a chilling message to scientists that vaccine safety and effectiveness is not to be investigated or questioned. They state this aggression makes vaccine safety science a "hazardous occupation".

Doctors also report being challenged by their own professional organizations when they question vaccine safety, report adverse events following vaccination, or write medical exemptions for their patients. The message is - "Don't question vaccines." [3]

"Recently, the authors of many vaccine safety investigations are being personally criticized rather than the actual science being methodologically assessed and critiqued. Unfortunately, this could result in making vaccine safety science a "hazardous occupation".

Critiques should focus on the science and not on the authors and on the scientists that publish reasonably high-quality science suggesting a problem with a given vaccine.

These scientists require adequate professional protection so there are not disincentives to publish and to carry out researches in the field. The issues for vaccine safety are not dissimilar to other areas such as medical errors and drug safety." [4]

These attacks are not unique to vaccines. We witnessed these same tactics with other health and safety concerns including:

- Smoking and lung cancer
- Mercury in dental fillings
- Fluoride in water
- Lead in gasoline and paint
- Food irradiation
- DDT and other pesticides
- Genetically Modified Organisms
- Thalidomide, Vioxx, Oxycontin

Immunization is a complicated topic that needs more reflection and less coercion. It's time to realize that vaccines, like medicines, are not a mystic panacea and that they are subject to the commercial and political pressure and also to the influence of conflicts of interest.

~ Dr. Claudina Michal-Teitelbaum, MD

18 Facts About Vaccines

The following are 18 facts about vaccines that every parent should be aware of:

Fact 1: Mandatory vaccination **violates the medical ethic** of informed consent, the Nuremberg Code, and the Universal Declaration of Bioethics and Human Rights.

Fact 2: The United States and Canada have **the most aggressive vaccine schedules** in the world. The number of recommended vaccines in the US and Canada have more than doubled since 1980. Children can receive as many as 53 doses of 15 vaccines by age 6. [1]

Fact 3: Canada is the only G7 nation without a national vaccine injury compensation program. [2] [3] If your child is injured by a vaccine in Canada, you are on your own.

Fact 4: The safety of the current CDC vaccine schedule has **never been proven** in large, long-term clinical trials. [4] [5] There is increasing evidence that the risks of vaccination outweigh the benefits.

Fact 5: Vaccines have **not been tested** for their ability to cause cancer, the degree to which a vaccine can damage an organism, their ability to damage genetic information, their ability to change genetic material, or for long-term adverse reactions. Product monographs make this fact clear. [6]

Fact 6: The current vaccine schedule has **never been tested for safety** in the real world way in which the schedule is implemented. [7]

Fact 7: No independent trials confirm the safety of giving multiple vaccinations at once. Research shows a dose-dependent association between the number of vaccines administered at the same time and hospitalization and death. [8]

Fact 8: No long-term clinical evidence exists that show vaccinated children have better overall health than unvaccinated children. [9][10]

Fact 9: There are **no clinical studies** that show injecting mercury into humans is safe. There is irrefutable evidence that the use of mercury in vaccine production increases the risk of neuro-developmental disorders. [11][12][13][14][15]

Fact 10: No clinical studies have been conducted to establish the safety of using aluminum in vaccines. The neurotoxicity of aluminum is well documented, affecting memory, cognition and psychomotor control, and causes damage to the blood brain barrier. [16]

Fact 11: The amount of aluminum used in vaccines **regularly exceeds the maximum** amount permitted by the FDA. [17] Two month old babies in Canada, the U.K., U.S and Australia are exposed to **49 - 54 times** the current safety limit for aluminum exposure.

Fact 12: Most vaccine safety trials use control groups consisting of other vaccinated populations or placebos containing aluminum. **These are not true placebos.** [18]

The failure of the pharmaceutical industry to use a neutral placebo undermines the integrity of CDC claims that vaccines have been proven to be safe and effective. [19]

Fact 13: The US Vaccine Court has awarded more than **3.7 billion dollars** in compensation for vaccine injuries and death since 1989. [20] This includes families whose children developed autism following vaccination. [21]

Fact 14: Artificially stimulated immunity via vaccines **is not life long**. Disease outbreaks regularly occur in fully vaccinated populations. [22] [23] [24] [25] The need for booster shots makes this self-evident.

Fact 15: Vaccine pre-license safety trials are not conducted by the government. They are conducted by the vaccine manufacturers who are immune from **liability** for the safety of their products.

Fact 16: Vaccine producers Merck and GlaxoSmithKline have **paid billions in criminal penalties** and settlements for research fraud, faking drug safety studies, failing to report safety problems, bribery, kickbacks, and false advertising. [26] [27]

Fact 17: The disclosures by CDC senior scientist, Dr. William Thompson, reveal the CDC has known for more than fifteen years that children receiving the MMR vaccine on schedule **are significantly more likely to regress into autism** compared with children whose parents decided to withhold the vaccine until the child was older. [28] [29] [30]

Fact 18: In the United States and Canada the rate of autism has increased from less than 1 in 10,000 prior to 1980 to more than 1 in 36 children today.[31] ADHD now affects 1 in 10 children.[32] [33] Genetic disorders do not evolve this quickly. An environmental influence is clearly indicated.

The greatest obstacle to discovery is not ignorance –
it is the illusion of knowledge.
~ Daniel Boorstin

Let's be clear: the work of science has nothing
whatever to do with consensus.
Consensus is the business of politics.
Science, on the contrary, requires only one
investigator who happens to be right,
which means that he or she has results that are
verifiable by reference to the real world.

In science consensus is irrelevant.

What is relevant is reproducible results.
The greatest scientists in history are great
precisely because they broke with the consensus.
There is no such thing as consensus science.
If it's consensus, it isn't science.
If it's science, it isn't consensus.
Period.

I regard consensus science as an extremely
pernicious development
that ought to be stopped cold in its tracks.
Historically, the claim of consensus has been
the first refuge of scoundrels;
it is a way to avoid debate
by claiming that the matter is already settled.

~ Michael Crichton, MD

Is the Delivery System Safe?

Vaccination is the infusion of contaminating elements into the system, and after such contamination you can never be sure of regaining the former purity of the body.

~ Dr. Alexander Wilder, MD
Professor of Pathology

Injecting Viruses is Unnatural

It's important for parents to understand that the practice of injecting viruses and foreign substances into the human body is unnatural.

The human body is not designed to encounter pathogens and toxins via intramuscular injection.

Infectious diseases are contracted through ingestion (swallowing) or inhalation (breathing). When vaccine ingredients are injected directly into the body they bypass the natural portals of entry and the normal protective filters, such as the lungs, digestive organs and skin.

This method of delivery permits the ingredients contained in vaccines, including mercury, aluminum, viruses, foreign DNA, and other toxic and harmful ingredients to enter the bloodstream, make their way into organs, bones and tissues, and cross the blood-brain barrier into the brain.

Vaccination amounts to a conjuror's trick, designed to accomplish by deception precisely what the whole immune mechanism has seemingly evolved to prevent – granting bacteria, viruses, and foreign antigens free and immediate access to the major internal organs of the immune system with no reliable means of getting rid of them.

~ Dr. Richard Moskowitz, MD

What Are the Ingredients in Vaccines?

If parents were provided with a list of vaccine ingredients, the list would include the substances below.

Did the medical authority that insisted your child be vaccinated show you this list prior to a shot? Mine didn't.

___

32

According to Dr Todd M. Elsner, this is what your child could receive in the first 6 years of his or her life: [1]

- 2-phenoxyethanol (antifreeze) – 17,500 mcg
- Aluminum (neurotoxin) – 5,700 mcg
- Fetal bovine serum – Unknown amounts
- Formaldehyde (embalming agent) – 801.6 mcg
- Gelatin (ground up animal carcasses) – 23,250 mcg
- Human albumin (human blood) – 500 mcg
- Mercury – unknown amounts
- Monosodium L-glutamate (causes obesity & diabetes) – 760 mcg
- MRC-5 cells (aborted human babies) – Unknown amounts
- Neomycin (antibiotic) – Over 10 mcg
- Polymyxin B (antibiotic) – Over 0.075 mcg
- Polysorbate 80 (carcinogen) – Over 560 mcg
- Potassium chloride (used in lethal injection to shut down the heart and stop breathing) – 116 mcg
- Potassium phosphate (liquid fertilizer) – 188 mcg
- Sodium bicarbonate (baking soda) – 260 mcg
- Sodium borate (for cockroach control) – 70 mcg
- Sodium chloride (table salt) – 54,100 mcg
- Sodium citrate (food additive) – Unknown amounts
- Sodium hydroxide (Corrosive) – Unknown amounts
- Sodium phosphate- 2,800 mcg
- Sodium phosphate monobasic monohydrate (toxic) – Unknown amounts
- Sorbitol (Not to be injected) – 32,000 mcg
- Streptomycin (antibiotic) – 0.6 mcg
- Sucrose (cane sugar) – Over 40,000 mcg
- Yeast protein (fungus) – 35,000 mcg
- Urea (metabolic waste – human urine) – 5,000 mcg

The CDC's repeated assurances that all of these ingredients are safe are hardly persuasive or even credible, since they have failed to provide any evidence of the slightest attempt to investigate them.

~ Dr. Richard Moskowitz, MD

Vaccines Contain Neurotoxins

Mercury: Vaccine manufacturers use mercury (Thimerosal) in the production of many vaccines, and as a preservative in multi-dose vials of the influenza vaccine. Mercury is recognized as the most toxic substance that is not radioactive.

The acceptable limit of mercury in drinking water in Canada is 1 parts per billion. In the US it is 2 ppb. A liquid with 200 ppb is considered toxic waste. Several brands of the infant influenza vaccine have 25,000 ppb. Many of the regular influenza vaccines have 50,000 ppb of mercury.

It is scientific fact that human brain neurons permanently disintegrate in the presence of mercury. There is no evidence injected mercury is safe in any amount. [2][3][4][5][6]

In fetuses, infants and children, low-dose exposure to mercury can cause severe and lifelong behavioural and cognitive problems. At higher exposure levels, mercury may adversely affect the kidneys, the immune, neurological, respiratory, cardiovascular, gastrointestinal, and haematological systems of adults. [7]

~ Canadian Medical Association

Aluminum: Aluminum is another neurotoxin used in vaccines. Aluminum has never undergone biological testing to determine whether it is safe. Aluminum, like mercury, was 'grandfathered' into our medical system without the benefit of safety testing.

Aluminum affects memory, cognition and psychomotor control and causes damage to the brain. Clinical evidence indicates aluminum is a primary etiological factor in dementia and Alzheimer's disease. Aluminum also interferes with gene expression and depresses mitochondrial function.

The amount of aluminum in many vaccines exceeds the maximum amount permitted by the FDA. [8][9]

A 2017 aluminum toxicity study conducted by Christopher Exley Ph.D., a world-renowned aluminum expert found:

Some of the highest quantities of aluminum ever recorded in the brains of autistic boys. [10]

Vaccines Contain Harmful Ingredients

Vaccines contain known neurotoxins, chemically altered viruses, antibiotics, preservatives, detergents, stabilizers, neutralizers, carrying agents, Polysorbate 80, MSG, formaldehyde, glyphosate, genetically modified viruses, and other harmful ingredients which counteract and/or bond synergistically thereby increasing their potential harm. [11] [12]

Mercury and other heavy metals adversely affect the gastrointestinal, immune, nervous and endocrine systems. Heavy metals alter cellular function and numerous metabolic processes in the body, including those related to the central and peripheral nervous systems. [13]

Vaccines Contain Animal DNA/RNA

Animals and insects are used in the manufacture of vaccines. Animals used include: monkey, cow, chicken, duck, pig, sheep, dog, horse, rabbit, guinea pig and mice.

The medium in which vaccine bacteria and viruses are cultivated include: rabbit brain tissue, dog kidney tissue, monkey kidney tissue, chicken or duck egg protein, chick embryo, calf serum and pig and horse blood. Animal tissues naturally contain animal DNA/RNA and viruses.

Animal viruses have the ability to implant their genetic material into the human genetic system. Animal proteins and viruses are foreign to the human body.

The animal DNA/RNA and viruses cannot be fully screened out during the manufacturing process.

Most vaccines are contaminated with a number of known and yet-to-be discovered viruses, bacteria, viral fragments and DNA/RNA fragments. Once animal DNA, viruses and retroviruses insert themselves into human cells, they cannot be removed. The injection of animal DNA/RNA compromises the biological integrity of the human race.

Unlike chemical pollutants which break down and become diluted out, retroviral nucleic acids are infectious, they can invade cells and genomes, multiply, mutate and recombine indefinitely.
Injecting animal viruses and retroviruses into humans is creating unknown new diseases and chronic illness. [14]

~ Dr. Judy Mikovits, Ph.D.

Vaccines Derived From Aborted Fetuses

Many live virus vaccines (measles, mumps, rubella, chicken pox, shingles) are grown in cell lines derived from aborted human fetuses. These include WI-38, cell cultures from a female fetus that was aborted in 1964, and MRC-5, cell cultures from a 14-week male fetus that was aborted in 1966. [15]

In addition to the clearly ethical and religious considerations of using aborted humans to grow vaccine viruses, these cell lines contain human DNA debris. Research indicates a causal relationship between vaccines manufactured using fetal cell-lines and the prevalence of autism spectrum disorder. [16]

Vaccines Affect Brain Development

During these early years, a baby's developing brain is particularly vulnerable to environmental toxic exposures. We recognize this with the risk of drinking alcohol during pregnancy. We know that cellular structures change rapidly during fetal growth and the early years, and that a toxic exposure at the wrong moment can permanently damage the brain.

> *One mistake early on, and the brain may be forever changed in subtle or serious ways.*
>
> ~ Dr. Philip Landrigan
> Dean for Global Health at Mount Sinai School of Medicine [17, 18]

It is not just toxic exposures from the external environment that threaten normal brain development. It's imperative we also recognize the risks of injecting highly inflammatory neurotoxic substances like aluminum into our infants during critical windows of brain growth.

Researchers are now discovering that aluminum adjuvants in vaccines can be transported into the brain and provoke ongoing chronic brain inflammation. With the current CDC vaccination schedule high quantities of aluminum are injected into an infant's fragile micro-environment during these highly sensitive early years of brain formation.

In the early years, in order to protect the developing brain during rapid brain growth, the baby's immune programming requires that it be in a non-inflammatory state. The key to insuring normal brain development is to protect the baby's immune system from anything that causes inflammation. [19]

If the immune system is provoked early on by inflammation, the normal course of brain development can be negatively impacted.

We now know that the brain has its own immune cells (the microglia), which play a crucial role in brain development. These immune cells are highly sensitive to inflammation. Vaccinations, by design, creates inflammation which then triggers the microglia to secrete highly toxic chemicals that can lead to a chronically inflamed state in the brain resulting in the destruction of connective synapses. [20, 21]

Immune activation triggered by infections or vaccines damage the growing brain.

This can result in life-long brain injuries, ADHD, mental illnesses, seizures/epilepsy, schizophrenia and autism. A large field of study has identified that cytokines, triggered by excessive immune activation, are involved in brain injury leading to autism. [22]

No clinical studies have been conducted to establish the safety of aluminum adjuvants in infants and children.

The scientists at *Vaccine Papers* extensively discuss the impact of inflammation on the brain during fetal and early life brain development. [22]

> *In particular, aluminum in adjuvant form carries a risk for autoimmunity, long-term brain inflammation and associated neurological complications and may thus have profound and widespread adverse health consequences.* [23, 24]

~ Chris Shaw PhD and Lucija Tomljenovic PhD., Neuroscientists

Approximately one-quarter of all children in the United States
now suffer from encephalopathy, autism, ADD, ADHD,
a learning disability, or some form of brain damage,
which the best contemporary science has shown to be largely,
if not entirely, autoimmune in nature.

There is now a solid body of evidence that not only the MMR
vaccine but also the other live-virus vaccines, as well as those
containing mercury, aluminium, and other adjuvants, are fully
capable of causing autoimmune dysfunction that regularly crosses
the blood-brain barrier and causes brain damage.

From these experiments it is only a short step to the inference
that autoimmune brain damage is well within the capacity
of every vaccine, and indeed an inherent property
of the vaccination process itself.

~ Dr. Richard Moskowitz, MD
Vaccines – A Reappraisal

Science is generated by and devoted to free inquiry: the idea that any hypothesis, no matter how strange, deserves to be considered on its merits. The suppression of uncomfortable ideas may be common in religion and politics, but it is not the path to knowledge; it has no place in the endeavour of science.

~ Carl Sagan

Many scientists are reluctant to consider . . . that their current theories may be wrong. This conservative stance is unscientific and is actually holding back progress.
The biggest hindrance to scientific progress is believing that a concept is true when it isn't.

~ Lee Bladon

Is Vaccine Science Trustworthy?

It is simply no longer possible to believe much of the clinical research that is published or to rely on the judgment of trusted physicians or authoritative medical guidelines.

~ Dr. Marcia Angell, MD
Editor - *The New England Journal of Medicine*

Science Has Been Corrupted

Pure science is a method of uncovering facts. The 'business of vaccination' has co-opted science and turned it into *'scientism'*. Scientism is a quasi-religious dogmatism that stifles critical thinking and acts on *blind faith* rather than the questioning that true science requires.

Much of the research on vaccines is not in discovery of the truth, but rather is in support of a prescribed agenda – universal vaccination. Vaccine science is not based upon principles of sound scientific methodology. Instead vaccine science is based on mystical claims of miraculous benefits.

Despite its ideals of objectivity, neutrality and collective benefit, vaccine science is grossly flawed with bias, prejudice and self-interest. When unchecked these biases influence funding decisions, who or what is studied, who has access to the research data, and who benefits from the results of scientific research.

> *We've missed ten years of research because the CDC*
> *is so paralyzed right now by anything related to autism.*
> *They're not doing what they should be doing*
> *because they're afraid to look for things that might be associated.*

~ Dr. William Thompson, CDC Senior Scientist

Real science is a noble venture, a quest for understanding through the honest evaluation of evidence. Science does not operate by consensus or belief. Science is never "settled". To state - *"the science is settled"* means they've abandoned science.

> *Genuine science welcomes challenges and debate*
> *and is open and transparent.*

We should be cautious of organizations like the CDC that respond to new information about vaccines as dangerous rather than welcome the development in our understanding.

When science is no longer in service to the truth, it is not science. It is medical industry propaganda.

It appears that our mission is being influenced and shaped by outside parties and rogue interests… and Congressional intent for our agency is being circumvented by some of our leaders. What concerns us most is that it is becoming the norm and not the rare exception. We are often directed to do things we know are not right.
These questionable and unethical practices threaten to undermine our credibility and reputation as a trusted leader in public health.

~ CDC Scientists Preserving Integrity, Diligence and Ethics in Research
August 29, 2016 [1]

Vaccine Herd Immunity Is Unproven

The promise of herd immunity is used to coerce legislators, doctors, public-health officials, medical personnel and the public into accepting forced vaccinations. What is not commonly known is that herd immunity is a *theory* based on *natural* infection, which in most cases provides lasting, long-term immunity.

The immune response stimulated by vaccines is temporary, lasting a few years or even as short as a few months. [2] There is insufficient evidence to conclude that artificial immune stimulation can ever create herd immunity.

The Tdap and MMR vaccines are good examples of the failure of vaccines to produce herd immunity. Based on the peer-reviewed published efficacy, at any given point in time only 5% of Americans have some sort of vaccine-induced immunity to pertussis, and 12% have full to half-immunity to measles. [3]

Dare to Question

The herd immunity we enjoy today is provided by the generations born before 1960 that experienced natural disease exposure. These individuals provide real herd immunity. Without the mantra of herd immunity, public-health officials and politicians would not be able to justify forced mass vaccinations and the loss of individual rights and freedoms.

If vaccinations worked as their proponents claim,
it wouldn't make any difference to the vaccinated
whether anyone else was vaccinated or not.

No parent should be pressured to vaccinate on the basis of speculation of vaccine induced herd immunity, or to risk his or her child's health in the hope it may protect someone else's child. The conflict between private and public rights contradicts the claims made by vaccination proponents.

Most Vaccines Don't Prevent Infection

What is also not commonly known is that most vaccines do not prevent infection or transmission of disease.

Five vaccines – polio, diphtheria, influenza, pertussis, and tetanus are not designed to prevent infection or transmission of disease. They are designed only to reduce the severity of symptoms should one become infected.

Four vaccine targeted diseases – tetanus, Hepatitis B, HPV, and Meningococus are not communicable through casual contact and therefore not easily transmitted.

Three of the vaccine targeted diseases – Pneumococcus, Influenza, and HPV have so many strains that vaccination does little to reduce the prevalence of the disease. Vaccination actually causes an increase in the strains not covered by the vaccine.

The fact is an individual who is not vaccinated with polio, diphtheria, tetanus, whooping cough, Hep B or Hib poses no extra danger to the public than a person who is. [4 5 6 7 8 9]

To imply that non-vaccinating individuals are a threat to the community is marketing propaganda, not evidence-based medicine. It is fear mongering, not science.

Vaccination Is an Uncontrolled Experiment

The gold standard of safety research compares a subject group with a control group. A true clinical trial utilizes a placebo – a substance that is known to be neutral or harmless.

Most vaccine safety trials use other vaccinated populations or placebos containing aluminum as the control group.[10] Neither of these are neutral placebos. In fact, not a single one of the clinical trials for vaccines given to babies and toddlers had a control group receiving a neutral placebo.

Vaccine safety trials that are conducted without a neutral placebo cannot determine if a product is safe.

Many pre-licensure trials do not include patient populations most at risk of serious adverse events. This is not responsible science. In fact, this is not science.

Vaccines given in the combination schedules recommended for our children today have never been tested for safety, which makes this practice a medical experiment. Vaccination is an uncontrolled experiment upon our infants and children.

Vaccine safety "science"
is not recognizable as science anymore.

~ James Lyons-Weiler, Ph.D.

The Claim That There is No Connection Between Vaccines & Autism Is Dishonest

It is unscientific and perilously misleading for the *Centre for Disease Control* to assert that vaccines and autism have been exhaustively studied and that no connection has been found.

While there are 16 or so industry-funded studies that are regularly cited by critics of the vaccine-autism hypothesis, these studies examine only one vaccine product (MMR) and one vaccine ingredient (Thimerosal).

It is illogical to exonerate all vaccines, all vaccine ingredients, and the total vaccine program based on a handful of epidemiological studies of just one vaccine product and one vaccine ingredient.

The studies used to deny a vaccine-autism link include the 2004 study which senior CDC scientist Dr. William Thompson revealed the CDC fraudulently withheld data with the express intention of misleading the public about the vaccine-autism link. This alarming disclosure is the basis of the 2016 documentary -*Vaxxed: From Cover-Up to Catastrophe.*

CDC funded studies conducted by Dr. Poul Thorsen used intentionally misleading data for the sole purpose of denying a link between vaccines and autism. [11] Thorsen is a wanted felon in the United States.

The remaining studies have been widely criticized in the scientific community for their lack of statistical power and design. None of the studies compares the rate of autism in an unvaccinated population with a vaccinated population. It would appear these studies were intentionally designed to not find a vaccine-autism connection. This is not science. This is propaganda masquerading as science.

——

Compelling Evidence that Vaccines Cause Autism

There is compelling evidence that a vaccine-autism connection exists:

There are now more than 144 independent research studies [12] that show a relationship between vaccination and autism. And more evidence is being uncovered every day.

A report in the *Pace Environmental Law Review Journal* reviewed 83 cases of vaccine-induced brain injury that resulted in an autism diagnosis, which were compensated by the U.S. Federal Vaccine Injury Compensation system. [13]

Award-winning journalist, Sharyl Attkisson, investigated the vaccine-autism link and compiled an extensive list of studies that show a vaccine-autism link - *What the News Isn't Saying About Vaccine-Autism Studies* – updated November 27, 2016. [14]

Attkisson concluded –

> *The body of evidence on both sides is open to interpretation. People have every right to disbelieve the studies on one side. But it is disingenuous to pretend they do not exist.*

Dr. Bernadine Healy, the former head of the *National Institutes of Health*, stated that the vaccine-autism link is not a "myth". Dr. Healy disclosed that her colleagues at the Institute of Medicine did not wish to investigate the possible link between vaccines and autism because of the impact they feared it would have on the vaccination program.

The failure to fully investigate the vaccine-autism link indicates the vaccine program is ideology and dogma rather than science.

It became clearer to me as I read the research, listened to more and more parents, and found other practitioners who also shared the same concern that vaccines had not been completely proven safe or even completely effective, based on the literature that we have today.

It didn't appear that the scientific studies that we were given were actually appropriately designed to prove and test the safety and efficacy.

It also came to my attention that there were ingredients in there that were not properly tested, that the comparison groups were not appropriately set up, and that conclusions made about vaccine safety and efficacy just did not fit the scientific standards that I was trained to uphold in my medical school training. [15]

~ Dr. Larry Palevksy, Pediatrician

Is Measles A Manufactured Crisis?

A few years ago a medical crisis was declared in Canada. The result was a tremendous outpouring of anger, resentment and judgment. People were called names. Consideration was given to removing a parent's right to make medical decisions for their children. Some even advocated for removing the children from those parents who didn't comply with the proclaimed action needed to ward off the impending medical crisis.

The crisis that triggered this outpouring of fear, anger and judgment – an outbreak of measles.

The media was incredibly vigilant in reporting every single case of measles. At last count there were 375 cases reported in British Columbia, 6 in Calgary, 1 in Edmonton, 11 in Regina and 11 in Ontario (*Huffington Post*, April 13, 2014).

Individuals of my generation are a bit mystified by the intensity of the purported crisis. As someone who grew up in the 1960's, everyone I knew contracted measles at some point in his or her childhood. Everyone also understood that getting measles in childhood provided long-term immunity. Now, a measles outbreak results in a reaction as intense as the SARS crisis of a few years ago, or the AIDS epidemic even prior.

How did this common and benign childhood event become so threatening that normally kind and well-intended individuals felt justified to treat others badly? How did measles become the basis for depriving individuals of their rights and freedoms?

Dare to Question

Two colleagues shared with me the impact of this purported crisis on their lives. One, the mother of a four year old, informed me that she finally succumbed to having her daughter vaccinated for measles after a barrage of phone calls day after day insisting that she *"do the right thing and get her daughter vaccinated." "You won't be able to live with yourself if your daughter gets measles,"* she was informed.

The second, another mother, shared with me the following:

"Hey, there's a measles outbreak! Have you heard? It's got just a wee bit of media attention. I'm having a difficult time filtering out the unkind things people have to say about people who do not vaccinate. Selfish. Should be kept in a bubble, sent to an island, and excluded from society. Stupid. Negligent. It's amazing how nasty people can be, and how it is apparently okay to be unkind about parental choices when the topic is vaccination."

I've received my own dose of unkind words and judgments when I've attempted to defend the rights of parents to make an informed decision regarding vaccination.

CTV News reporter Jon Woodward holds people like me responsible for the reduction in vaccination rates in his commentary – 'BC Vaccination Rates Drop Amid 'Misinformation campaign'. Woodward is typical of most media pundits in his assessment that I am the one who is "misinformed". Woodward's failure to provide or demand any evidence of the safety and effectiveness of the measles vaccine is not considered relevant.

The *National Post* conducted a survey to elicit opinions on whether vaccinations ought to be mandatory and thus deny a parent the right and responsibility to choose what is in their children's best interest.

Not surprisingly, given the bias in the media's reporting of this complex topic, the majority of Canadians responding to this survey supported denying a parent the right to make this medical decision.

This event is similar to numerous other events in recent years. Witness the reporting on 9/11 and the need for an invasion of Iraq and Afghanistan. We were inundated with information that was purported to be true by well-informed 'experts'. Remember those weapons of mass destruction? Some kind of urgent action is needed, we were told. There is no time to think. There is no time to discuss the matter. Anyone who does not respond as demanded is irresponsible, selfish, delusional and dangerous.

Psychologists understand how it is that we are so easily coerced into a reactive response. They describe the process as 'Problem – Reaction – Solution'. A problem is manufactured. A reaction is elicited. And a solution is offered. Witness the recent events: measles outbreak = crisis = this is terrible and something must be done = take away a parent's right to voluntary, informed consent.

We would be wise to be more discerning in how we can be coerced into making reactive decisions rather than thoughtful and well-informed decisions. We ought to be especially sensitive to situations where we are emotionally hijacked, then told an immediate action is needed without the benefit of thoughtful discourse. These reactive actions undermine our capacity to use our gifts of intelligence and compassion.

We all deserve better. The answer will not be in the way mainstream media reports these issues. Rather the answer will be our unwillingness to become easily manipulated and coerced into supporting a reactive response.

Dare to Question

In this fear-based scenario, the questioning voice of reason is drowned out amid the hysteria surrounding the emerging 'killer infections', which are such a favorite media topic.

The propagation of fear by the media and by its sources in the public health industry has resulted in a growth of power in this industry far beyond the usual checks and balances of our democracy. [1]

~ Dr. Philip F. Incao, MD

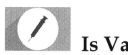 # Is Vaccine Policy Sound?

Any possible doubts, whether or not well founded,
about the safety of the vaccine cannot be allowed to exist.

~ Federal Register. Vol 49, No 107.

The Federal Register is the official journal of the Federal government of the United
States that contains government agency rules, proposed rules, and public notices.

Vaccination Distorts Public Health Priorities

Vaccination shifts public health priorities from effective and natural interventions like clean water, closed sanitation, improved hygiene, reduced exposure to toxins, clean air, better housing, breastfeeding, good nutrition and quarantine.

These public health measures were responsible for the significant decrease in mortality and the increase in health in the last century, not vaccinations. Quarantine was very effective during small pox epidemics.

Public health agencies are ignoring these effective health measures and have mistakenly identified 'increased vaccine uptake' as the desired outcome rather than 'improved health'.

When trying to achieve any goal,
it is important to measure the correct outcome.
Our goal should be improved health.

Vaccination Policy is Anti-science

Vaccination has become politicized such that honest debate is no longer permitted. The active censorship of concern about vaccine safety, effectiveness and necessity eliminates an important safeguard and increases our vulnerability to being harmed.

Stating that, "All vaccines are safe and effective" is like saying "All prescription drugs are safe and effective". Such statements are without scientific integrity and are meaningless. In the vaccine science domain much of what claims to be science is not scientific at all. Censoring discussion about vaccine safety, effectiveness and necessity is anti-science and anti-democracy.

___

54

Vaccination Is Not a Medical Issue

Vaccination is not a medical issue. Rather vaccination is a financial and ideological issue disguised as a medical issue.

If vaccinations were truly a medical issue there would be more interest in whether vaccines were safe, whether they prevented the targeted illnesses, and whether the health of those receiving vaccines was better than those who did not.

The reality of the vaccine program becomes evident when we witness the amount of financial and human resources dedicated to promoting vaccines and tracking vaccine compliance, rather than tracking vaccine safety and effectiveness.

The virtual absence of interest in vaccine safety and effectiveness is a strong indication that the intention of the vaccination program is not improved health.

Vaccine Policy Undermines Rights and Freedoms

Vaccine policy violates our rights and freedoms as citizens and erodes our parental rights and responsibilities to make medical decisions for our children.

Efforts to increase vaccine compliance include coercion, financial incentives and disincentives, punishment, restriction to education, childcare and employment, even imprisonment.

If the State can tag, track down and force individuals to be injected with biologicals of known and unknown toxicity today, then there will be no limit on which individual freedoms the state can take away in the name of the greater good tomorrow.

~ Barbara Loe Fisher

Dare to Question

Mandatory vaccine policy is a clear and direct violation of the Nuremberg Code, developed in response to the medical experimentation conducted by the Nazis, as well as a violation of the Universal Declaration on Bioethics and Human Rights; Article 6 – Consent: [1]

Any preventive, diagnostic and therapeutic medical intervention is only to be carried out with the prior, free and informed consent of the person concerned, based on adequate information. The consent should, where appropriate, be expressed and may be withdrawn by the person concerned at any time and for any reason without disadvantage or prejudice.

Vaccine mandates should only be considered if:

    1) A disease has a high rate of mortality.
    2) The disease is highly contagious.
    3) The vaccine is proven to be safe.
    4) The vaccine is effective in preventing transmission.

None of the current diseases and vaccines meets these criteria.

Vaccine Policy Ignores Individual Variables

The vaccine paradigm utilizes a 'one-size-fits-all' approach. Vaccine dosage is not calibrated by age, weight, immune response, gender, genetics, medical or family history, or other variables used to discern safe levels of a medical intervention. In no other area of medicine are individual variables systematically ignored.

This mandatory one-size-fits-all approach to vaccination is a de facto state-sanctioned selection of the genetically and biologically vulnerable for sacrifice.

~ Barbara Loe Fisher

Vaccines Are A Class of Drugs

Vaccines are referred to as if they are a single drug rather than a class of drugs. Vaccines vary by ingredients, manufacturer, purpose and method of action. No two vaccines work the same.

To lump all vaccines together irrespective of disease or vaccine type (live attenuated, inactivated whole cell, split virus, high dose, low dose, adjuvanted, monovalent, polyvalent) is irresponsible. To speak of vaccines as if they are one product is marketing propaganda.

No Individual Risk-Benefit Consideration

The decision whether to vaccinate or not ought to be evaluated on a disease-by-disease basis, a vaccine-by-vaccine basis, and an individual-by-individual basis. The merit of a vaccine ought to be determined by taking into consideration the risk of getting the disease, the consequences of getting the disease, the effectiveness of the vaccine, and the safety of the vaccine for the individual.

Universal vaccination is not science.
It is ideology.

All vaccines are not created equal.
Discussion of both the benefits and the risks
of individual vaccines is needed.
The authoritative medical bodies must end their arrogant stance
and take an honest look at the literature they have suppressed.
Negative effects must be honestly brought to light.
Legislative bodies need to do their homework and reject any thought
of mandating vaccinations.

~ Dr. Ralph Campbell, MD

Vaccine Promotion Relies On Fear & Ignorance

Vaccine promoters utilize fear and ignorance rather than informed consent in their efforts to increase vaccine uptake. Their goal is a compliant citizenry, not a consenting public.

Vaccine advocates show little regard for the medical ethic of informed consent. Rather, fear mongering and hysteria are the tools commonly used to promote universal mass vaccination. In the US, hospital personnel are reporting parents who refuse to vaccinate their newborn to Child Protective Services. This is effectively medical kidnapping and extortion.

Measles is an example of the current hysteria and fear mongering promulgated by public health entities, the pharmaceutical industry, and a corporate controlled media. The fact is measles is a harmless illness in healthy and well-nourished children. In first-world countries an individual is much more likely to die from the measles vaccine than from contracting measles.

Deaths in the U.S. during the past 10 years:
2004 to 2015

Due to Measles

Due to Measles Vaccines

ZERO

108

Source: CDC

Source: VAERS database

The fear mongering by public health, the pharmaceutical industry and the corporate media is dishonest and dangerous.

Any action that is dictated by fear and coercion of any kind ceases to be moral.

~ Mahatma Gandhi

Is the Claim of Safety Valid?

*The current science doesn't allow for an informed understanding
of an individual's genetically determined risk
for an adverse event due to a vaccine.*

~ Dr. Gregory Polland, MD
Vaccine Research Group – Mayo Clinic

Vaccine Adverse Events

Adverse events reported following vaccination: [1]

- Autism
- Asthma
- Immune system dysregulation and dysfunction
- Seizure disorder
- Neurological deficits
- ADD/ADHD
- Learning disabilities
- Life threatening allergies
- Obesity
- Brain injury
- Coma
- Guillain-Barre Syndrome
- Cancer
- Chicken pox
- Shingles
- Polio
- Encephalopathy
- Mental retardation
- Motor and sensory deficits
- Brain inflammation
- Chronic nervous system dysfunction
- Anaphylaxis
- Febrile seizures
- Brachial neuritis
- Arthritis
- Smallpox, polio, measles and varicella zoster vaccine strain infection
- Shock and unusual shock-like state
- Protracted, inconsolable crying
- Sudden Infant Death (SIDS)
- Death

Vaccination Disregards the Hippocratic Oath

The first principle of medicine is – 'First do no harm'. In 2011 the United States Supreme Court concluded that vaccines are - *"unavoidably unsafe"*. This means health officials inject substances into our infants, children and adults which they know can cause significant harm and death.

Following the medical precautionary principle,
the default position for vaccination must be recommendations,
not compulsion. Compulsion, not only undermines trust,
but limits the fundamental rights to life, liberty, bodily integrity,
informed consent, privacy, and to parental decision-making.

~ Mary Holland, JD
NYU School of Law

Doctors are unable to predict which of us will be seriously harmed or die from vaccination.

The US Vaccine Injury Compensation Program has awarded more than $3.7 Billion for vaccine injury since 1989. [2]

Every G7 Nation, excepting Canada, has a national vaccine injury compensation program. These Nations recognize vaccines cause injury and death and compensate for significant injury and death.

Vaccines can't be both "safe" and "unavoidably unsafe".

No Evidence Vaccinated Individuals Are Healthier

The *Journal of Translational Science* published the first independent, non-industry funded study comparing the overall health of vaccinated and unvaccinated 6 to 12 year old children in the United States. [3]

The results of the study reveal that while vaccinated children were significantly less likely to have chicken pox or whooping cough, they were significantly more likely to have pneumonia, allergies, otitis media (ear infection), eczema, a learning disability, Attention Deficit Hyperactivity Disorder (ADHD), Autism Spectrum Disorder, neuro-developmental disorders, and chronic illness.

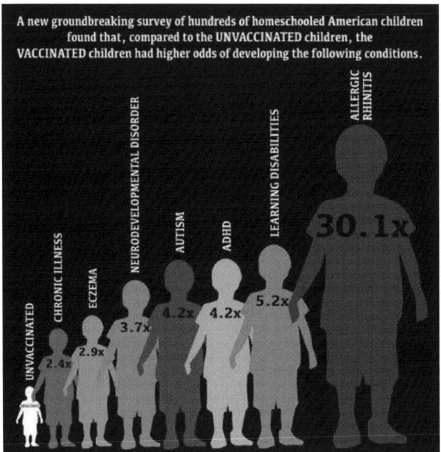

Graphic from Children's Medical Safety Research Institute (CMSRI)

No significant differences or benefits were seen with hepatitis A or B, measles, mumps, meningitis (viral or bacterial), influenza or rotavirus.

A 2012 vaccine study reported a linear relationship between the number of vaccine doses administered at one time and the rate of hospitalization and death. [4]

The results also showed that the younger the infant at the time of vaccination, the higher the rate of hospitalization and death.

The safety of CDC's childhood vaccination schedule was never affirmed in clinical studies. Health authorities have no scientific data from synergistic toxicity studies on all combinations of vaccines that infants are likely to receive.

National vaccination campaigns must be supported by scientific evidence. No child should be subjected to a health policy that is not based on sound scientific principles and, in fact, has been shown to be potentially dangerous. [5]

~ Neil Z. Miller

There is no substantive evidence that children receiving the current vaccine schedule are healthier than those who don't.

Vaccine Manufacturers Not Accountable for Safety

Many parents are not aware that the vaccine industry in the United States is not legally liable for the safety of their products. The vaccine industry was granted legal immunity by an act of the US Congress in 1986. The nuclear industry is the only other industry that is not legally responsible for the harm their products cause.

The result of this legal immunity is that no one can be held responsible for the injuries and deaths caused by vaccination.

This freedom from liability includes not only the vaccine manufacturers, but also government agents in the CDC and FDA, and those who encourage, license and administer vaccines including doctors and nurses.

A consequence of this legal immunity is there is no legal or financial incentive for the pharmaceutical industry to make vaccines safer, even when there is evidence that vaccines can be made safer. This creates a very dangerous situation. **The vaccine industry has effectively been given license to injure and kill with impunity.** There is evidence that the legal immunity provided to vaccine manufacturers has increased the risk of harm. [6]

This legal immunity was not designed to protect citizens. It was designed to protect the pharmaceutical industry.

It's nothing but hubris that allows scientists to ignorantly think they can imitate natural immunity by injecting scores of foreign substances into human beings to raise targeted antibody levels without disrupting or destroying cells, tissues, systems, and processes.

~ Brent Wilcox
Author of *Jabbed*

Vaccine Schedule Not Tested for Safety

One of the major criticisms of the vaccine industry is its failure to conduct long-term clinical trials that prove the safety of the current vaccine program. [7][8][9]

The prestigious *Institutes of Medicine* (IOM) found that the safety of the current childhood vaccine schedule has never been proven in large, long-term clinical trials:

Few studies have attempted more global assessment of entire sequence of immunizations or variations in the overall immunization schedule and categories of health outcomes, and none has squarely examined the issue of health outcomes and stakeholder concerns in quite the way that the committee was asked to do its statement of task. None has compared entirely unimmunized populations with those fully immunized for the health outcomes of concern to stakeholders. [10]

Vaccines have not been tested for the ability to cause cancer (carcinogenicity); the ability to damage an organism (toxicity); the ability to damage genetic information within a cell (genotoxicity); the ability to change the genetic information of an organism (mutagenicity); the ability to impair fertility; and for long-term adverse reactions.

Most vaccines currently on the market have been approved based on studies lasting only a few weeks or days. [11]

For a vaccine to be administered without adequate safety data is nothing short of medical malpractice.

Adequate human data on use during pregnancy are not available.

~ DTP product insert

Vaccination Increases Infant Death

A study comparing the rate of vaccination with the rate of infant mortality in first world countries identified a relationship between the number of vaccines given in the first year of life and the rate of infant mortality. The more vaccines given, the higher the rate of infant death. [12] The United States and Canada have a higher rate of infant mortality than some third world countries.

The United States, which vaccinates newborns and has the most aggressive vaccination schedule in the first year of life in the world, has the highest infant mortality rate of any developed country in the world. [13][14] Canada, which is second in the number of vaccines given in the first year of life, is ranked 28th in infant mortality (2009 infant mortality rates).

In an urban African community, a study found that the DTP vaccine is associated with a five-times higher mortality than children unvaccinated with DTP. No study has shown beneficial survival effects of the DTP vaccine. [15]

In July 2017, the U.S. Court of Federal Claims ruled that there was "preponderant evidence" supporting the claim that vaccines "actually caused or substantially contributed" to Sudden Infant Death Syndrome (SIDS). [16]

Multiple Vaccine Exposure Increases Risk

The current vaccine schedule recommends multiple vaccine injections at one time. In nature, the human body is not subject to multiple disease agents, toxic chemicals, foreign DNA and retroviruses at one time.

There are no studies examining the synergistic effects of giving multiple injections at once.

Exposure to multiple infectious agents and the accompanying toxic ingredients via injection increases the likelihood of a compromised immune system, making the infant more vulnerable to illness, serious adverse reactions and death. [17]

Multiple injections place an unnatural and unnecessary burden upon the immune system and compromise its ability to work effectively. Every new vaccine added to the schedule increases the complexity and the risk of adverse reactions.

Are Vaccines Effective?

Vaccination at its core is neither a safe nor effective method of disease prevention.

~ Tetyana Obukhanych, Ph.D.
Immunologist

Evidence of Effectiveness Is Not Required

Most individuals lose their elevated antibody levels two to ten years after being vaccinated. Approximately ten percent of the population has no increased antibody response to a vaccine. At any given time a significant portion of the population has no increased antibodies to the diseases they had been vaccinated against. The absence of disease outbreaks begs the question of whether vaccines are necessary.

Vaccine manufacturers are not required to demonstrate vaccines actually reduce the rate of disease contraction, contagion, complication or mortality. It is simply assumed that elevated antibody levels equate to immunity, despite the lack of supporting evidence.

Vaccines are the only medication where evidence of effectiveness and absence of harm are not required before approval. This is especially evident with the HPV vaccine.

There is no clinical evidence the HPV vaccine
has prevented anyone from contracting cervical cancer.

Vaccine efficacy ought to be evaluated based on clinical evidence the vaccine actually increased disease prevention and improved health. This does not occur with the vaccine program.

Vaccines Spread Disease

Live-virus vaccines spread disease through viral shedding. Live-virus vaccines include: measles, mumps, rubella, nasal flu, shingles, rotavirus, chicken pox, oral polio and yellow fever. [1] Vaccine strain live-virus can be shed in body fluids such as saliva, nasal and throat secretions, breast milk, urine and blood, stool and skin lesions.

Shedding after vaccination may continue for days, weeks or months depending on the vaccine and the individual.

Vaccinated individuals risk spreading disease every time they are re-vaccinated. Vaccinated individuals can also be infected, yet remain asymptomatic thereby unknowingly spread the disease. Viral shedding is the reason recently vaccinated individuals are not permitted to visit hospital wards of cancer and immune suppressed patients.

Vaccines Eliminated Herd Immunity

The vaccine program has effectively eliminated herd immunity. Vaccinated individuals do not have life-long immunity to infectious diseases. In the developed world, herd immunity no longer exists and hasn't since the 1960s. The vaccination program has extinguished the widespread herd immunity that benefited the majority of people due to natural exposure to measles, mumps, whooping cough, rubella and chicken pox.

The introduction of mass vaccinations has drastically changed the natural and safe pattern of disease experience.

Infants were protected from diseases by maternal immunity. Adults were protected by their own permanent immunity, which nearly all of them acquired in their childhood via the disease experience. Mild childhood diseases have now been pushed into infancy and adulthood where they have more serious consequences.

Vaccines do not protect us for a lifetime. They only postpone the susceptibility to the corresponding infection rather than extinguish the susceptibility completely. No one knows when the vaccine's protective effect expires. This uncertainty increases the risk of contracting 'vaccine preventable diseases'.

Dare to Question

Vaccination Increases the Risk to Infants

Vaccination reduces the maternal antibody protection transferred from a mother to her newborn. [2] [3] The result is the infant of a vaccinated mother is more at risk of infectious disease earlier in life than the infant of a mother with naturally acquired immunity.

Disrupting the natural cycle of the mother-infant immunity transfer is a dangerous and irreversible consequence of prolonged vaccination campaigns. The vaccine paradox is that while vaccines may reduce the incidence of disease in childhood, they put the next generation of infants more at risk.

Humanity is now dependent upon artificial immune stimulants for temporary protection.

This dependence results in three critical health concerns. Firstly, vaccination has created universal drug dependence that is less effective than the natural maternal antibody protection. Secondly, the many adverse effects of vaccines lead to numerous health consequences. Thirdly, vaccines have pushed childhood diseases into infancy and adulthood.

Vaccination Interferes With Immune Development

The maturation of the immune system is accomplished by learning how to mount an acute, vigorous response to an infection. Childhood diseases such as measles, mumps, chicken pox, influenza and other infectious diseases are considered 'challenge illnesses' that prime and develop a child's immune response. Recovering from a childhood illness is *"the formative experiences by which good health is achieved and maintained."* [4] Vaccination removes this significant evolutionary step from a child's immune development. The long-term effect of this is unknown.

70

Measles is known to have a protective effect against many diseases including cancer, heart disease, malaria, allergic diseases, and juvenile rheumatoid arthritis. Developmental leaps have been observed in children following measles. Chicken pox exposure reduces the incidence of shingles in adults. Mumps helps prevent ovarian cancer. [4]

Dr. Richard Moskowitz, a physician with more than fifty years of clinical experience, has concluded that the artificial suppression of disease by vaccination is detrimental to our overall health and well being.

Vaccination Causes New Strains to Emerge

Vaccines cause microbes, bacteria and viruses to mutate. This can result in the growth of disease strains that are more severe and resistant to current medical treatments. We witnessed this phenomenon with the excessive use of antibiotics.

Haemophilus influenza B is an example of a disease that was effectively suppressed by vaccination. Other serogroups, however, rose to displace the strain suppressed by the vaccine. The same phenomenon occurs with the HPV vaccine. Thus the need to continually add more strains to the vaccine.

In response to mass pertussis vaccination campaigns in the 1950s, the B. pertussis microbe evolved to evade both whole cell and acellular pertussis vaccines, creating new strains producing more toxin to suppress immune function and causing more serious disease. This is the primary reason for the outbreak of pertussis today.

The rapid altering of disease strains via vaccination may actually put humanity more at risk of a pandemic infection to which our immune systems are not able to respond.

Anti-bodies Do Not Equal Immunity

The CDC claims that, *"Immunity to a disease is achieved through the presence of antibodies to that disease."* The CDC deems a vaccine to have efficacy solely on the basis that it increases antibody levels in the blood. Research, however, demonstrates that an individual can have immunity with low or no antibodies, while others can become infected even when antibody levels are high.

Our immune response is significantly more complicated than the level of antibodies in our blood.

Vaccines Compromise Health

Good health is dependent upon a healthy body and a strong immune system. The injection of multiple antigens, adjuvants, toxic and foreign matter can overwhelm the immune system and impede its ability to fight infection. Immunologists have expressed concern that the growing number of vaccines given early in life may impair immune function for life.

Studies show a dose dependent relationship between the number of influenza vaccines received and susceptibility to a pandemic virus. [5] A 2017 study revealed that women who had received the H1N1 influenza shot and then received a normal influenza vaccine were 7X more likely to have a spontaneous abortion. [6]

Vaccination is essentially an artifice, designed to trick the immune mechanism into providing a semblance or counterfeit of immunity that is partial, defective, and temporary at best, and that carries substantial additional risks of its own.

~ Dr. Richard Moskowitz, MD

Is Vaccine History Accurate?

It is pathetic and ludicrous to say we ever vanquished smallpox with vaccines when only 10% of the population was ever vaccinated.

~ Dr. Glen Dettman, Pathologist

Vaccine Impact is Dishonest

The pharmaceutical industry and mainstream media routinely refer to vaccines as *'a miracle of modern medicine'*, a distinctly unscientific term. Vaccines are consistently described with no conditions or qualifiers and an absence of supporting evidence.

Vaccines are regularly credited with the reduction in the mortality of infectious diseases, the elimination of small pox and polio, and having saved millions of lives. The historical and scientific evidence does not support such claims.

While some vaccines have suppressed the incidence of some infectious diseases, the significant reduction in mortality and the improved health in the last century occurred <u>before</u> the introduction of vaccines. Diseases like scarlet fever and the plague were eliminated without the benefit of any vaccine. Giving vaccines credit for the elimination of infectious disease and the decline in mortality is a myth, albeit a popular one.

Contrary to popular belief, vaccines did not eliminate either small pox or polio. [1] [2] There is substantial evidence these early vaccines actually contributed to an increase in both diseases and caused more injury than the disease itself. [3]

During the 'polio epidemic' in the 1950s, every case of paralysis was deemed to be caused by the polio virus. We now know that most of the paralysis was in fact not caused by the polio virus. Scientists now recognize that other viruses like Coxsackie, echo and enteroviruses caused paralysis, as did exposure to neurotoxins such as lead, arsenic and DDT.

Poliovirus infection, even during the peak epidemic, was a low-incidence disease that was falsely represented by the pharmaceutical industry as a rampant and violent crippler.

Paralytic conditions still exists today. The World Health Organization has simply relabeled the paralysis as *Acute Flaccid Paralysis*. In 2012, India reported 60,292 cases of acute flaccid paralysis. Indian doctors have observed that 'non polio acute flaccid paralysis' increases with the number of doses of oral polio vaccine distributed in the country. [4]

Prior to the discontinuation of the oral polio vaccine in the US, the oral polio vaccine caused all cases of polio.

When one gets the history wrong, this leads
to getting our public health priorities wrong.

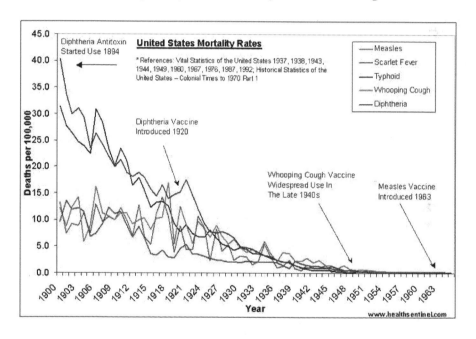

The best evidence offered by those promoting (vaccines)
is that there has been a reduction in the incidence of certain diseases
against which vaccination is now commonplace.
This is not evidence.

~ Dr. Vernon Coleman, MD

Vaccine Safety Claims Are Dishonest

The medical industry consistently makes the unqualified claim that vaccines are *"safe and effective"*. How can vaccines be "safe and effective" when more than $3.7 billion has been paid in compensation for vaccine injury in the United States?

In addition, the vaccine industry has been forced to withdraw more than 32 vaccines from the US market because of the ineffectiveness or harm these vaccines caused. [5] The list of withdrawn vaccines includes: small pox, swine flu, DPT, MMR, rotavirus, and oral polio vaccines, among others.

The polio vaccine given to 100 million Americans during 1955-1963 was contaminated with a monkey virus known as SV 40. SV40 causes cancer in humans. It is now widely recognized that the polio vaccine contributed to the significant increase in cancers we experience today. [6]

The Vaccine Industry Distorts the Risk of Disease

The vaccine industry greatly exaggerates the risk of contracting diseases targeted by vaccines. The true potential of a vaccine ought to be assessed based on the number of people who developed a serious complication following infection, rather than the infection itself. What is rarely discussed in vaccine promotion literature is the rate of serious complications in the pre-vaccine era. The rate of serious complications in the pre-vaccine era were as follows: [7]

Measles – In the years preceding the introduction of the measles vaccine in 1963 the death rate from measles in the US population was 1 in 500,000 people.

Mumps – Prior to the mumps vaccine in 1967, about 1 in 4 million people in the US population died from mumps.

Chicken pox - In the population as a whole, prior to the introduction of the chicken pox vaccine, 1 in 2.3 million Americans died of complications from chicken pox each year.

Rubella - The fatality rate prior to the widespread use of the rubella vaccine in 1969 was 1 person in 9 million in the US population. The rate of birth defects in pregnant women was about 1 in 20,000 births.

Hib - Before the Hib vaccine was introduced in 1985 about 1 in 2 million people in the U.S. population died annually from meningitis. The risk of permanent harm from meningitis was about 1 in 600,000 in the US population.

Rotavirus - Prior to the vaccine being introduced in 2006 about 1 in 10 million in the U.S. died from rotavirus.

Polio - Before widespread use of the vaccine in 1955 the permanent paralysis rate or death from polio in the U.S. population was 1 in 100,000 people.

The Rate of Serious Illness in Children Today: [8] [9]

Attention Deficit Hyperactivity Disorder - 1 in 10 children
Learning Disability - 1 in 6 children
Mental Illness - 1 in 30 children
Allergies - increased 6X since 1980
Anaphylactic Food Allergies - doubled in the last decade
Eczema - 1 in 5 children
Asthma - 1 in 8 children
Seizure Disorder - 1 in 20 children
Autism - 1 in 36 children [10]
Sudden Infant Death - the leading cause of infant death

We and our children have been and are the victims of a
carefully orchestrated, programmed propaganda campaign
in which maximum publicity is repeatedly given
to rare complications from one of the childhood diseases
while actively suppressing
the cases of morbidity and death caused by vaccines.

This active suppression is used to quietly terrorize any professional
who does honest research and reports negative or adverse effects
from mandated vaccines.

~ Dr. Thomas Stone, MD
Pediatrician

How to Manufacture Consensus

The world is a complex and complicated place. It's impossible for each of us to understand and evaluate all that is presented to us on a daily basis. In our effort to manage the complexities of life we take short cuts. We trust. We trust in the wisdom and integrity of others to inform us on matters that we are unable to research and evaluate for ourselves.

When the trust is honestly earned and has integrity the trust can serve us well. It releases us from the burden of figuring everything out for our self and allows us to focus our attention and energy in specific areas of interest and passion. Unfortunately, our trust in institutions, organizations and authority is being eroded because honesty and integrity is being sacrificed in the interest of profit and power.

At one time we could rely on the declaration that consensus was reached. Consensus is a powerful tool that is regularly used to reassure us that a particular perspective or course of action has been well researched, discussed, debated, and a conclusion reached based on solid evidence. Efforts are made to reassure us by the power of consensus whether the issue is the safety of genetically modified organisms, the validity of climate change, the safety and effectiveness of vaccinations, the quality and integrity of industrial safeguards, or even the need for war.

Unfortunately, according to Jon Rappoport, author of *The Matrix*, the process of consensus building has become much less collaborative and evidence-based and is more often *"manufactured."*

The manufacture of consensus looks like the following:

1. An 'authority', often unnamed, declares an idea or a perspective as fact.

2. Respected individuals, groups, governmental organizations and the media repeat the authoritative message over and over as if it is fact.

3. The position is taken that because consensus has been reached further discussion and debate is no longer needed or tolerated.

4. Critics and dissenters of the consensus position are attacked. Shock and dismay is expressed that there are *"still people who refuse to accept the obvious."*

5. Warnings are issued and dire consequences predicted if everyone does not accept the consensus idea or perspective.

6. Carefully constructed 'scientific' studies are produced to support the consensus position.

7. A declaration is made that the consensus idea or position represents 'the greatest good for the greatest number'.

8. Legalized coercion through the introduction of new laws and regulations is introduced to prevent anyone from holding or expressing a dissonant opinion or position.

9. Any dissenter is relegated to the margins and dismissed with labels that deny them a voice or any credibility regardless of their experience or stature.

10. Eventually no one can recall a time when the original idea was seriously disputed.

Science once offered us confidence that a statement, fact or conclusion was true based upon a rigorous and verifiable process using the scientific method. This is an accepted method to produce verifiable data that will serve in the best interests of truth. Unfortunately the scientific method, a process of hypothesis, data collection, analysis and confirmation or refusal of the hypothesis has been corrupted.

Where once we could trust the scientific method, today science is being co-opted for economic and political gain and is no longer a valid seal of approval.

Science, like other aspects of our society,
has been corrupted by power and politics.
It is no longer in service to the truth.

Rather, it is in service to those in positions of power and who have enough money to determine the outcome of 'science'.

Consider these two quotes from editors of prestigious science/medical journals:

It is simply no longer possible to believe much of the clinical research
that is published or to rely on the judgment of trusted physicians
or authoritative medical guidelines.
I take no pleasure in this conclusion, which I reached slowly and
reluctantly over my two decades as an editor
of the New England Journal of Medicine.

~ Dr. Marcia Angell, MD

The case against science is straightforward:
much of the scientific literature, perhaps half
may simply be untrue.
Science has taken a turn toward darkness.

~ Richard Horton
Editor in Chief, Lancet

Rappoport explains that these efforts to manufacture consensus are effective because people have a minimal tolerance for conflicting views on subjects of key importance. He believes humans are wired for consensus.

While consensus is certainly desirable, the question is whether the consensus is based on solid, supported evidence, and whether the good that is being promoted is indeed for the greater good or whether the consensus has been manufactured for the benefit of a small group of individuals or organizations.

We need to be more discerning of whether the consensus is worthy of our respect.

> *Who is the individual or group declaring consensus?*
> *Is there integrity in their decision-making process?*
> *Is there a willingness to let the science speak?*
> *Is there investment in a particular outcome?*
> *Are there economic, political or strategic interests that can compromise the integrity of the decision?*
> *Is there independent access to the supporting data?*
> *Are we giving away our responsibility for decision-making to those who have not earned our trust?*
> *Are we unduly influenced by the authority of government, the medical community and the media?*
> *Are we willing to think for ourselves?*

We would be wise to be cautious in accepting consensus positions when other motives are involved that can corrupt a true consensus process.

> *When an organization uses marketing propaganda instead of science, there is a reason.*

Can Vaccine Oversight Be Trusted?

*The combined and cumulative effects of 55 shots, 209 vaccine antigens,
525 mcg of mercury and 13,425 mcg of aluminum that have been injected
into a child by 18 years of age in accordance with the CDC's
2017 childhood immunization schedule has never been examined.*

In fact, it has never even been questioned.

~ Dr. David Brownstein, MD

Doctors Not Taught to Recognize Vaccine Injury

Doctors receive no formal training on how to diagnose or treat vaccine injury. Absent from current medical school curriculum is complete and up-to-date information about vaccine ingredients, diagnosis and treatment of vaccine injury, adverse events reporting, and individual genetic susceptibilities to vaccine injury.

The harm this causes is significant. A doctor's failure to recognize and report vaccine injury puts other children at risk for the same fate. Their failure to acknowledge vaccine injury also discourages the development of safer vaccines or alternative methods of immune support and disease prevention.

The reporting of vaccine injury is essentially voluntary as there are no consequences for failing to report vaccine injury. A Harvard Medical School study found that less than 1% of vaccine adverse reactions were reported. [1]

A doctor's inability to recognize vaccine injury prevents families from getting the help they need. A doctor's inability to acknowledge vaccine injury undermines informed consent. Informed consent is only as informed as your doctor is informed.

The CDC Admits To Limited Knowledge of Risks

According to the CDC's website, [2] the Institute of Medicine (IOM) concluded that *"there are limitations in our knowledge of the risks associated with vaccines"*. The IOM identified the following problems:

1. *Limited understanding of biological processes that underlie adverse events.*

2. *Incomplete and inconsistent information from individual reports.*
3. *Poorly constructed research studies.*
4. *Inadequate systems to track vaccine side effects.*
5. *Few experimental studies were published in the medical literature.*

CDC policies and decisions directly affect vaccine policies in nations worldwide. It's important to question why various governments are mandating vaccines when so little is known about the long-term impact of universal mass vaccination.

Wisdom is knowing how little we know.

~ Socrates

Vaccine Producers Pay Billions in Penalties

Every US manufacturer and supplier of pediatric vaccines has pled guilty to fraud in the last four years.

Vaccine producers Merck and GlaxoSmithKline have paid billions in criminal penalties and settlements for research fraud, faking drug safety studies, failing to report safety problems, bribery, kickbacks and false advertising. [3] [4]

There are two active whistleblower cases in the US Federal Court against Merck alleging scientific fraud with regard to their claims of the safety and effectiveness of the MMR vaccine.

Do not think it worthwhile to produce belief
by concealing evidence,
for the evidence is sure to come to light.

~ Bertrand Russell

The CDC Has Conflicted Interests

The *Center for Disease Control* has conflicted interests. The CDC is responsible for monitoring the safety of vaccines, and at the same time they have a mandate to increase vaccine uptake. The CDC is both a regulatory agency and a major corporation in the vaccine industry.

Most people are unaware the CDC is effectively a for-profit corporation. The CDC holds patents on over 50 vaccines and sells more than $4.5 billion worth of vaccine products each year. Acknowledging concerns about the safety of vaccines would negatively affect their revenues.

Federal conflict of interest rules do not apply to the CDC. Those responsible for licensing vaccines routinely benefit from the sale of vaccines. We shouldn't have to wonder if those in the CDC are acting in the public's best interest or their own.

It is difficult to get a man to understand something when his salary depends upon his not understanding it.

~ Upton Sinclair

Vaccine Producers Not Accountable to the Public

The vaccine industry is projected to be a $59 billion industry by 2020. [5] Its goal, like all businesses, is to have the highest financial return possible. They do this by eliminating competition, using advertising and propaganda to promote their products, and they employ lobbyists to influence governments. According to Robert Kennedy Jr., the pharmaceutical industry has four times as many lobbyists in Washington as the military-industrial complex. The vaccine industry is not accountable to the public. They are only accountable to their shareholders. Profit is what matters.

Inadequate Post Marketing Monitoring

The post-marketing monitoring of vaccine products is grossly inadequate. One problem is that the monitoring of vaccine safety is passive rather than active. A passive system only recognizes a tiny percentage of vaccine adverse events. The real number of children and adults experiencing vaccine injury is unknown.

A second concern is that medical professionals receive no formal training on how to recognize vaccine adverse events or report vaccine injury.

Public information related to vaccine safety is inadequate
to enable parents and governments
to make informed vaccine decisions.

Thirdly, vaccine producers do not know the long-term impact of the current vaccine schedule on our neurological and immune systems. [6] This is because vaccine producers are not required to conduct long-term safety studies. Most safety studies last a few weeks. Some are as short as a few days. [7]

Fourthly, vaccine producers are not required to conduct vaccinated vs. unvaccinated studies to prove that vaccines are safe and effective. Vaccine producers are able to market their products with less safety testing and oversight than is required with any other pharmaceutical drug.

Finally, there is substantial evidence that the CDC has repeatedly committed scientific fraud in its vaccine safety studies. This is particularly true with studies examining the role of vaccines in the autism epidemic. [8] Without proper monitoring and oversight the whole premise of vaccination safety, effectiveness and necessity is speculation rather than evidence based.

Abuse of Mature Minor Doctrine

The 'mature minor doctrine' is a term for the statutory, regulatory or common law policy, which accepts that a minor may possess the maturity to choose a particular health care treatment without the knowledge or agreement of his or her parents. This policy, incorporated into various Health Acts in Canada and the United States, was originally intended to allow adolescents to freely access birth control and abortions.

Schools and public health agencies now use this doctrine to coerce children as young as eleven to consent to vaccination without parental knowledge or consent. A document from the *Canadian Teachers Federation* lauds the cost effectiveness of the school vaccination platform and the power of leveraging the authority of schools and threat of suspension to pressure students to 'consent' to vaccination.

Children are told that they can sign their own consent form without consulting his/her parents. Rarely are these children told that they have the legal right to vaccine exemptions; that vaccination, like any medical treatment is voluntary; nor are they provided with adequate information on vaccine risks. This means that real informed consent is being denied.

Vaccination Clinics Don't Belong in Schools

Vaccination clinics held in school cafeterias are an exercise in herding students through a process as quickly as possible. Students are not given privacy to voice medical concerns. The practitioners providing the injection often have no knowledge of the student's medical or family history. And the simple act of rolling up one's sleeve is deemed evidence of consent. It is clear that protocols to insure that the consent of minors is informed and voluntary are inadequate.

Can Vaccine Journalism Be Trusted?

Dr. Peter Doshi, Associate Editor for the *British Medical Journal* (BMJ) made the following statements about good journalism as pertains to vaccinations:

"Good journalism on this topic will require abandoning current practices of avoiding interviewing, understanding, and presenting critical voices out of fear that expressing any criticism amounts to presenting a "false balance" that will result in health scares.

If patients have concerns, doubts, or suspicions − for example, about the safety of vaccines, this does not mean they are anti-vaccine.

Approaches that label anybody and everybody who raises questions about the right headedness of current vaccine policies as "anti-vaccine" fail on several accounts.

Firstly, they fail to accurately characterize the nature of the concern. Many parents of children with developmental disorders who question the role of vaccines had their children vaccinated . . . and people who have their children vaccinated seem unlikely candidates for the title.

Secondly, they lump all vaccines together as if the decision about risks and benefits is the same irrespective of disease − polio, pertussis, smallpox, mumps, diphtheria, hepatitis B, influenza, varicella, HPV, Japanese encephalitis − or vaccine type − live attenuated, inactivated whole cell, split virus, high dose, low dose, adjuvanted, monovalent, polyvalent, etc.

Dare to Question

This seems about as intelligent as categorizing people into 'pro-drug' and 'anti-drug' camps depending on whether they have ever voiced concern over the potential side effects of any drug.

Thirdly, labeling people concerned about the safety of vaccines as 'anti-vaccine' risks entrenching positions. The label (or its derogatory derivative 'anti-vaxxer') is a form of attack. It stigmatizes the mere act of even asking an open question about what is known and unknown about the safety of vaccines.

Fourthly, the label too quickly assumes that there are "two sides" to every question, and that the "two sides" are polar opposites. This "you're either with us or against us" thinking is unfit for medicine.

Contrary to the suggestion — generally implicit — that vaccines are risk free (and therefore why would anyone ever resist official recommendations), the reality is that officially sanctioned written medical information on vaccines is — just like drugs — filled with information about common, uncommon, and unconfirmed but possible harms.

Medical journalists have an obligation to the truth.

Its time to listen—seriously and respectfully—to patients' concerns, not demonize them."

All truth passes through three stages.
First, it is ridiculed.
Second, it is violently opposed.
Third, it is accepted as being self-evident.

~ Arthur Schopenhauer
German philosopher (1788 – 1860)

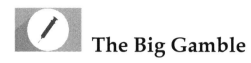 # The Big Gamble

If the public were ever to lose confidence in vaccination,
it would mark the beginning of the end of the medical establishment
as we know it today.

~ Dr. Robert Mendelsohn, MD

The vaccine industry, including the government agencies mandated with the responsibility for vaccine oversight is gambling.

They are gambling that the best way to preserve public confidence in the vaccine program is to deny and disavow any claims that vaccines have a role in the serious adverse events that are routinely witnessed following vaccination.

Rather than investigate every act of injury or suspected harm as occurs in other industries, most notably the airline industry and the food industry, the vaccine industry has adopted the mantra of "safe and effective" and "vaccines do not cause autism". Their official position is – 'the science is settled' and 'no further research is needed'.

Any possible doubts, whether or not well founded,
about the safety of the vaccine cannot be allowed to exist.

~ Federal Register. Vol 49, No 107 June 1, 1984

When the number of recommended vaccines and the number of reported adverse events was low, this strategy held a high likelihood of success. The number of injuries was not significant enough to capture the attention of the mass consciousness.

As the number of recommended vaccines has grown from a handful to 69 doses of 16 vaccines by the age of eighteen the number of children injured or killed by vaccines has reached epidemic proportions. 1 in 6 has a chronic neurological or immunological condition. The house of cards that forms the basis of the vaccine paradigm is faltering.

It is a well-known fact in toxicology that contaminants exert a mutual synergic effect, and as the number of contaminants increases, the effects grow less and less predictable. With each new vaccine added to the recommended schedule the complexity of drug interactions and the mounting toxic load increases the certainty of a collapse.

A wise and safety conscious industry would evaluate the risk of collapse and carefully manage the number of vaccines injected into children. They would know that a system based on trust can dissolve overnight as occurred with the dot.com bubble and the financial and housing meltdown of 2008.

But the vaccine industry is not wise.
It is not safety conscious.

It sees only unlimited potential for growth and profit. It has been lulled into complacency and the illusion of invulnerability by the 1986 Act of Congress, which relieved the vaccine industry of all legal liability for the safety of their products.

This lack of legal liability and accountability, the assurance of a captured and expanding market due to government imposed mandates, and the lack of any real investigative journalism by the 'not so free press' has produced a climate of exponential growth that is too attractive and financially rewarding to resist.

—

Instead of being committed to producing safe and effective products, the vaccine industry is in a race to produce as many vaccines as possible while lobbying corruptible governments to increase mandates for school attendance, daycare, housing and employment.

How many of the 270 vaccines currently under development will be mandated is anyone's guess given the present consciousness.

What the vaccine industry hasn't taken into consideration is that parents are waking up to the harm that is being done to their children. Parents whose children have been permanently harmed or killed by vaccines are refusing to be coerced into subjecting their children to more vaccines. They are 'mad as hell and are not going to take it anymore'.

These parents are refusing to be intimidated into silence by a captured and compliant corporate media. The chants of "correlation does not equal causation" mean little when your once healthy child is experiencing uncontrolled seizures or requires 24-hour care for the rest of his or her life.

The outcome of this uncontrolled experiment is not in doubt. The blind faith and unearned trust in the vaccine program and its high priests will come to a sudden and dramatic end. The vaccine industry will collapse under the weight of its own fraud, immorality and callous disregard.

The only question is how many more children, teenagers and adults will be injured or killed by vaccines before the awareness is substantive enough to cause this teetering structure to fall.

The collapse will be swift.

Like the housing market in a faltering economy and stocks in a financial meltdown, soon the vaccine industry will not be able to give their products away. Vaccines will be avoided like the plague they were intended to protect us from. And whatever good was hoped for by the architects of the artificial immunization program will be lost for generations as trust, once abused will be difficult, if not impossible to reclaim.

The vaccine industry could have avoided this collapse but they were too greedy and too callous in their disregard for those injured by their products.

I suggest the collapse has already begun. The once revered medical industry is losing its appeal, and the growing awareness of massive vaccine injury can no longer be contained.

Thankfully, the end is near.

A mass vaccination program carries a built-in temptation to oversimplify the problem; to exaggerate the benefits; to minimize or completely ignore the hazards; to discourage or silence scholarly, thoughtful and cautious opposition; to create an urgency where none exists; to whip up an enthusiasm among citizens that can carry with it the seeds of impatience, if not intolerance; to extend the concept of the police power of the state in quarantine far beyond its proper limitation; to assume simplicity when there is actually great complexity; to continue to support a vaccine long after it has been discredited; (and) to ridicule honest and informed consent.

~ Statement from Clinton R. Miller
Intensive Immunization Programs, May 15th and 16th, 1962.
Hearings before the Committee on Interstate and Foreign Commerce House of Representatives,
87th Congress, second session on H.R. 10541.

10 Unanswered Questions

There are a number of questions we ought to be asking and demanding answers to regarding the medical practice of artificial immune stimulation:

1. Is it reasonable or responsible to continue to inject human beings, particularly infants and pregnant women with mercury and aluminum, which are known neurotoxins?

2. Why is it that we don't hold those individuals recently vaccinated with a live virus (chicken pox, measles, mumps, rubella, intranasal influenza, shingles) responsible for the spread of diseases due to viral shedding?

3. Should the U.S. Center for Disease Control be trusted on issues of vaccine safety given one of their own senior scientists, Dr. William Thompson, has come forth alleging scientific fraud and the destruction of data that was supported at the highest levels?

4. Is the breadth and depth of studies done on the safety of the current vaccine schedule adequate given the research is done by those with a financial conflict of interest?

5. Have the children who have gotten sick, disabled or died from vaccine reactions been extensively studied to identify their vulnerabilities or the vaccine's defects? Isn't it important to identify vulnerable children or the vaccine's limitations in order to prevent further tragedies and loss of life in the future?

6. Do we have a responsibility to those children, their families and potential vaccine victims to conduct independent vaccine safety studies?

7. How many children are we willing to sacrifice in pursuit of the theory of 'herd immunity' or 'the common good'. Who decides which child's life is worth sacrificing?

8. Why has only one independent long-term clinical study been conducted that compares the health of vaccinated vs. never vaccinated individuals? Why have the results of this study not been made publicly available?

9. Why is the low incidence of autism in non-vaccinated children not a serious matter of investigation by the CDC, and why is this important fact rarely reported by the mainstream media?

10. Why is discussion about this controversial medical practice actively discouraged by governments, the media, and vaccine manufacturers?

"There is a great deal of evidence to prove that immunization of children does more harm than good.

~ Dr. J. Anthony Morris
Former Chief Vaccine Control Officer, FDA

Where Do We Go From Here?

If we can all agree that our goal is to have healthy children with strong immune systems, then we need to recognize that vaccinations aren't taking us where we want to go.

Any one of the more than 45 concerns listed in this document is substantive enough to question the validity of the artificial immune stimulation program. Collectively they provide compelling evidence that the vaccine program is a flawed and dangerous experiment. Vaccines are not as safe, effective or necessary as we have been led to believe.

Vaccinated children are not healthier
than unvaccinated children.

Vaccinology is dogma and ideology masquerading as science. The extent of harm this ideology is causing is unfathomable. It's time to end this arrogant and unscientific mass injection of toxic chemicals and infectious matter into our children.

- √ Vaccine mandates must end.
- √ Liability protection of manufacturers must end.
- √ Voluntary informed consent must be upheld.
- √ Independent and verifiable evidence of vaccine safety and effectiveness must be produced.

It's time to respect and nurture our natural ability to fight infection and to sustain health. Modifying or delaying a flawed vaccination program is not the answer.

Unless we change our direction,
we will end up where we are headed.

~ Chinese proverb

Dare to Question

The denial of informed consent must end.
The systematic misinformation campaign to lure parents into
vaccinating their children against their instinct must end.
The enrollment - without consent - of millions of men, women and
children in vaccine experiments must end.

Mandates are not the answer.
Individualized medicine is the answer.
Science is the answer.
Persecuting fraud is the answer.
Putting an end to pseudoscience on vaccine safety issues
is the answer.
Ending pseudo-skepticism is the answer.

~ James Lyons-Weiler Ph.D.
President, Institute for Pure and Applied Knowledge

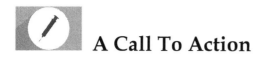# A Call To Action

The vaccine issue is more than about health. It is also about human rights. If we do nothing, our rights and freedoms will continue to be eroded and eventually eliminated.

We will lose our right to informed consent and self-determination. We will lose the right and responsibility for medical decision-making for our children. Our access to education, employment, housing, daycare, volunteerism, travel, and government services will be increasingly restricted.

As responsible and conscious parents and citizens, it's imperative that we claim our rights and responsibilities. This requires more than simply educating ourselves about vaccine injury. What is needed is a 'call to action'. I invite you to consider engaging in the following activities and actions:

1. Educate yourself on the risks and dangers of universal mass vaccination.

2. Join a vaccine choice advocacy organization and support its efforts. A listing is below.

3. Reach out to other parents and family members. Share what you have learned with others.

4. Develop your own 'network of support'. Questioning the current 'consciousness' on vaccination can be isolating. Find others who will support you.

5. Meet with your government representatives. Demand full and unfettered choice pertaining to the medical practice of vaccinations.

6. Demand the repeal of the 1986 National Childhood Vaccine Injury Act in the United States.

7. Demand that vaccine manufacturers be held legally liable for vaccine injury and death.

8. Demand that the results of all vaccine clinical trials be made public.

9. Demand independent, vaccinated vs. unvaccinated studies to determine the risks and benefits of universal vaccination.

10. Speak loudly and firmly. Refuse to be silenced.

This is a critical time in our evolution as a society. It's time to claim our power and responsibility as sovereign citizens.

*What kind of society do you want to leave
for your children?*

Vaccine Choice Advocacy Organizations

Canada:
Vaccine Choice Canada   wwww.vaccinechoicecanada.com

United States:
National Vaccine Information Center - www.nvic.org
Stop Mandatory Vaccinations -
www.stopmandatoryvaccinations.com
World Mercury Project - www.worldmercuryproject.org
Physicians for Informed Consent
        https://physiciansforinformedconsent.org

Two Kinds Of Parents

There are two kinds of parents who come to Vaccine Choice Canada.

One group of parents recognizes they have a right and a responsibility to make an informed decision about the medical practice of vaccinations. These parents, prior to the birth of a child or even pre-conception, thoughtfully engage in educating themselves about the risks and benefits of vaccination.

Admittedly the number of parents who proactively engage in the vaccine decision is small. Given the overwhelming intensity and uniformity of the messaging by the medical industry and the magnification of these messages in the mainstream media, it is unusual for a young parent to question the safety, effectiveness and necessity of vaccines and thus engage in any real self-education.

By far the majority of parents who contact Vaccine Choice Canada are parents who trusted the direction of their doctor. They believed that the 12 vaccines given in 26 doses in the first 12 months of life (Ontario recommendations) were all safe, effective and necessary, only to witness significant injury or regression following the vaccination of their child.

A once content baby is suddenly inconsolable. A walking infant is now unable to stand. A talking child is now silent. An alert and attentive baby becomes unengaged. Instead of a happy, content and healthy child these parents suddenly have a child with agitation, poor attention, diarrhea, rashes, allergies, lethargy, and seizures.

Dare to Question

Some children go on to develop autoimmune diseases, immune system and neurological injuries, and some tragically pass away as mine did.

Something Is Wrong

Even though their Doctor tells these parents that any relationship between a vaccine and injury, disability or death is simply a "coincidence", these mothers and fathers know better. They know something is terribly wrong with their child.

The child they knew prior to the vaccinations is gone.

This is when many parents reach out to Vaccine Choice Canada. This is when the serious investigation of a vaccine's ingredients, adverse effects, and the pursuit of information on vaccine safety and effectiveness begin in earnest.

This awakening of parental concern *after* a vaccine injury is, unfortunately, all too common. Most of us at Vaccine Choice Canada are parents who willingly and naively subjected our children to the dictates of the medical industry, only to discover that vaccines were not safe and effective for our child.

Their first task is to find what treatments might heal their injured child. Who is knowledgeable about vaccine injury? How can these heavy metals be removed? How do I heal a leaky gut? How do I restore health? How do I support a compromised immune system? How do I undo the neurological damage that has been done?

Sometimes answers are found and their child makes a full recovery. Often times the damage is irreversible.

After having attended to their ailing child and having done all they can to recover as much health and capacity as possible, many of these parents begin a new journey. They take on a new focus and passion. They become advocates for informed consent.

They want other parents to know the risks and dangers of the current artificial immunization program. They want other parents to avoid the mistake they made. They want the medical industry to be held accountable for their actions and their unsafe products. They want the mainstream media to tell the truth about vaccines.

Mad As Hell

These parents begin the difficult journey of being labeled as *"anti-vaxxers, irresponsible parents, lunatics, celebrity chasers, unscientific and ignorant"*. But the blame and shame from a misinformed society and captured mainstream media do not deter them. They know the truth. They are not *"vaccine hesitant"*. They are *"mad as hell and not taking it any more"*.

No amount of shaming, threatening, cajoling, punishment or fake science will silence them or convince them of the safety and effectiveness of the universal, "one size fits all" artificial immune stimulation program. These informed parents will only accept solid, verifiable evidence of vaccine safety and effectiveness, which even a modest review of the vaccine literature reveals a disturbing absence of.

The absence of real scientific evidence of vaccine safety and effectiveness leads informed parents to conclude the vaccination paradigm is ideology rather than evidence-based medicine; and more akin to religion than science. Parents whose children have been harmed no longer accept the vaccine ideology on faith. Their trust has been broken.

Dare to Question

Welcome to informed consent. Welcome to the thinking mom and dad's revolution. Welcome to Vaccine Choice Canada. Together we will be warriors for truth, accountability and integrity. Together we will make the world safer for all children. Together we will protect and preserve our rights to informed consent and security of the person. Together we will uncover the truth, even if it is too late for our children.

Vaccine Choice Canada was formed in response to growing parental concern regarding the safety of current vaccination programs in Canada.

Our Mandate is:

- To empower parents to make an informed decision when considering vaccines for their children.

- To educate and inform parents about the risks, adverse reactions, and contraindications of vaccinations.

- To respect parental choice in deciding whether or not to vaccinate their child.

- To provide support to parents whose children have suffered adverse reactions and health injuries from childhood vaccinations.

- To maintain links with groups similar to ours around the world through an exchange of information and research, thereby empowering parents to reclaim health care choices for their families.

- To support people in their struggle for health freedom and to maintain and further the individual's freedom from enforced medication.

VCC publishes two issues of the Journal annually as well as a bi-monthly E-Bulletin.

If Not Vaccines, Then What?

If not vaccines, then what can we do to protect our infants and children? How can we ensure that they develop a strong immune system and normal brain growth?

Breastfeeding

Without question, the most important protective measure is breastfeeding. Breastfeeding provides optimal protection to your infant during the first two years of life. This is the period when the brain and immune system are rapidly growing.

New parents are not told that they already have access to the most effective immunological protection and brain enhancement for their baby. Breastfeeding provides the perfect food to insure the best health outcome, which will serve your child for life.

Breast milk is so exquisitely refined that it continually changes and adapts to the baby's needs as they change. Breast milk provides the infant brain with the specific micro-nutrients needed to insure optimal neural development and intelligence.

Breastfeeding endows the child with a living immune system capable of protecting the baby from many infectious diseases. It is a living fluid, rich in immune cells, which engulf and destroy pathogens and provides the baby with the appropriate and specific antibodies to fight infections.

Breast milk contains stem cells that can repair invisible harms that may occur during illness, high fevers, and vaccine-induced injuries.

Dare to Question

Nature has provided breastfeeding as a sophisticated living immune system, which responds to pathogens the baby is exposed to and provides specific antibodies and protective enzymes. Breast milk is constantly changing, responding to the baby's developmental needs and stages of growth.

When mothers breastfeed their infants, they can be confident they are providing their babies with the finest balance of nutrients for optimal brain growth complimented by unparalleled immune system protection.

For more information on the benefits of breastfeeding, download the '**New Parent Guide**' from Vaccine Choice Canada. [1]

Natural Means of Disease Prevention

Vaccine marketing has distracted attention and effort away from natural means of disease prevention and health promotion including clean air and water, good hygiene and nutrition, reducing exposure to toxins, and quarantine when needed.

Below is a summary of some of the natural and effective immune supports that have been ignored or minimized in the single focused promotion of vaccine products.

Clean Water

Researchers Cutler and Miller identified that clean water is critical to disease prevention and to the decline in infant mortality. In their 2004 paper [2] they concluded:

Our results also suggest that clean water was responsible for 3/4 (74%) of the decline in infant mortality and nearly 2/3 (62%) of the decline in child mortality.

*The magnitude of these effects is striking. Clean water
also appears to have led to the near eradication of typhoid fever
[and other] scourges such as pneumonia, tuberculosis,
meningitis, diphtheria/croup.*

*Clean water technologies are likely the most important
public health intervention of the 20th Century.*

If governments were really concerned about health, they would be using their resources to ensure that all citizens in the world have access to clean water.

Building Natural Immunity With Food

The following information has been contributed by Sally Fallon Morell. Sally is the founding president of *The Weston A. Price Foundation* and author of the best-selling cookbook *Nourishing Traditions*. Sally is also the author of *The Nourishing Traditions Book of Baby & Child Care*.

"The decision not to vaccinate does not mean that parents can be careless about protecting their children from disease. While some of the illnesses we vaccinate for are extremely rare (tetanus, diphtheria), unlikely to cause harm to children (chicken pox, mumps, rubella) or not a threat to children (hepatitis B), others like measles or polio can have serious consequences in poorly nourished youngsters.

It's up to parents to provide the kind of diet that will give their child robust natural immunity — that's the same kind of diet that will give a child good health overall. It's also a diet that can help your child recover from vaccination injuries.

Here's a list of recommendations to keep your children healthy and strong:

Foods Rich In Vitamin A

Vitamin A is our number one protection against disease. The immune system cannot function without vitamin A. Two important points about vitamin A:

- First, we cannot get adequate vitamin A by converting the carotenes in fruits and vegetables into the true vitamin A.

- Secondly, vitamin A requires vitamins D and K2 as co-factors. Foods that provide us with vitamin A, usually also contain vitamins D and K2 — foods like butter from grass-fed cows, egg yolks from pastured chickens, aged natural cheese, shellfish and organ meats like liver.

In addition to these foods, cod liver oil can provide vitamins A and D on a daily basis.

Before the advent of vaccinations, the medical profession knew that the vitamin A in cod liver oil would protect children against all sorts of infections.

Moms are recommended to take cod liver oil while pregnant and nursing, and to begin giving it to their children around two or three months. Use only cod liver oil containing natural vitamins. (See westonaprice.org/cod-liver-oil/ for more information and product recommendations)

Raw Milk

Raw milk is a complete, highly digestible food for growing children. It is also a powerful immune builder. A key component of our immune system is antibodies, such as immunoglobins, which are found in raw milk.

Vaccines are supposed to work by stimulating the production of antibodies, but babies cannot make antibodies, including vaccine-induced antibodies, until they are at least one year old. Yet babies today get over a dozen vaccines before the age of one.

Babies get antibodies from their mother's milk, or from the milk of another species. In fact, raw milk—whether human, cow, goat, sheep, camel, reindeer or water buffalo—contains all the components of blood except for red blood cells.

Raw milk creates the immune system in the infant, and nourishes that immune system throughout the period of growth. All of these valuable immune components, however, are destroyed by the heat of pasteurization.

Studies from Europe indicate that children who drink raw milk have fewer respiratory infections and less asthma, allergies and skin rashes compared to children who do not consume raw milk. (For more information, and to find raw milk, visit realmilk.com.)

Fermented Foods

Fermented foods like raw sauerkraut, homemade kefir and aged raw cheese contain beneficial protective bacteria. Eaten on a daily basis, the bacteria in these foods colonize the intestinal tract where they provide powerful protection against pathogens.

During the past twenty years, scientists have learned that gut bacteria are critical to health. In fact, about 80 percent of our immune system comes from beneficial gut flora. In addition, the biofilm of good bacteria in the gut provides a barrier to heavy metals like aluminum and mercury.

Avoid Processed Foods

In this age of industrial food production it's difficult to avoid processed foods, but parents will confer the great blessing of good health on their children by keeping them away from processed food. Especially avoid refined sweeteners like sugar, high fructose corn syrup and agave. Sugar uses up nutrients that the body needs to support the immune system.

Vegetable oils are also known to depress the immune system, while natural saturated animal fats support the immune system. Cook in animal fats like butter and lard, and give your children butter instead of margarine and spreads. Make your own salad dressing using olive oil rather than purchase ready-made dressings, which are made with the cheapest oils and loaded with additives.

In short, the recipe for protecting your children from disease and ensuring they will grow up healthy and strong is an old-fashioned, home-prepared diet rich in butter, eggs, cheese and nutrient-dense animal foods like liver and red meat. Fruits and vegetables can serve as vehicles for butter and cream!

The addition of raw milk, fermented foods, bone broths and, above all, cod liver oil to your child's diet will compensate for the occasional junk food that cannot be avoided. This is the Wise Traditions diet—vastly superior than vaccinations for protecting your children from disease throughout their growing years."

For further information: www.westonaprice.org

When diet is wrong, Medicine is of no use.
When diet is correct, Medicine is of no need.

~ Ayurvedic Proverb

How To Minimize Vaccine Injury

If you must vaccinate, you can reduce the risk of vaccine injury in your children with the following guidelines:

1. Consider delaying as long as possible. Some medical doctors recommend waiting at least two years until the child's immune system is more developed.

2. Breastfeed your infant. Breastfeeding provides your infant with a sophisticated living immune system, which responds to pathogens that your child may be exposed to.

3. Give large doses of Vitamin C to your child before any vaccination. This will help to reduce the negative side effects.

4. Never vaccinate your child when he or she is sick.

5. Refuse any vaccine that uses mercury as a preservative.

6. Request vaccines with the lowest aluminium content.

7. Refuse to allow your child to receive multiple vaccines at once. Request single dose vaccines.

8. Space out the shots to allow you to monitor your child's response to each vaccine.

9. Don't continue to vaccinate if your child has a reaction to a shot. Educate yourself on what vaccine adverse events may look like.

10. Request and read the product information insert for each vaccine. Don't rely on your doctor to inform you of the risks and contraindications.

11. Find a doctor who respects your questions and your concerns.

12. Consult with a Naturopath. Investigate homeopathic remedies and other immune supports. Homeopathic remedies can reduce the injury caused by vaccination.

13. Trust your intuition. If it doesn't feel right, don't do it. No one knows your child better than you do.

14. Do not be pressured into vaccinating your child simply because it's the "recommended schedule".

15. The fewer vaccines, the better. Research shows the risk of injury increases with the number of vaccines given and the earlier they are given.

16. Know your rights. Become a member of a vaccine choice advocacy organization. Most jurisdictions have exemptions for medical, religious and personal belief.

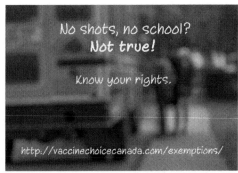

(Image courtesy of Vaccine Choice Canada)

Where Can I Get More Information?

Below is a short list of books, DVDs and online resources to assist you in becoming better informed on vaccine issues:

Books

Vaccines – A Reappraisal
- Richard Moskowitz MD

A truly wonderful book on why the vaccine process, by its very nature, imposes substantial risks of disease, injury and death that have been persistently denied by the vaccine industry, vaccine policy makers and the medical profession. It is without a doubt, the most important book on this topic that has been published in many years. Dr. Moskowitz draws on 50 years of general medical practice caring for children and adults.

Vaccine Safety Manual
- Neil Z. Miller

This bestselling guide to common childhood illnesses and vaccines evaluates each vaccine for safety, efficacy, and long-term effects. Impeccably researched and referenced, it contains the most comprehensive, up-to-date, uncensored data available – information that many doctors don't even know. In addition, health alternatives are offered, along with legal options to mandatory shots.

Dissolving Illusions
- Suzanne Humphries MD, and Roman Bystrianyk

Dissolving Illusions details facts and figures from long-overlooked medical journals, books, newspapers, and other sources. Using myth-shattering graphs, this book shows that vaccines, antibiotics, and other medical interventions are not responsible for the increase in lifespan and the decline in mortality from infectious diseases.

Vaccine Illusion
- Tetyana Obukhanych Ph.D.
In the debate over vaccine safety we have lost sight of a bigger problem: how vaccination campaigns wipe out our herd immunity and endanger the very young. Written by an immunologist, Vaccine Illusion explains why vaccines cannot give us lasting immunity to infectious diseases and how they jeopardize our natural immunity and overall health.

Vaccine Epidemic
- edited by Louise Kuo Habakus, and Mary Holland, JD

Vaccine Epidemic focuses on the searing debate surrounding individual and parental vaccination choice. Public health officials state that vaccines are safe and effective, but the truth is far more complicated. Coercive vaccination policies deprive people of free and informed consent - the hallmark of ethical medicine. Polls show that public concern about vaccine safety is increasing, and the right to make voluntary, informed vaccine choices. This is an essential handbook for the vaccination choice movement and required reading for all people considering vaccination for themselves and their children.

Saying No to Vaccines
- Dr. Sherri J. Tenpenny MD
This most comprehensive guide explains how and why vaccines are detrimental to you and your child. Dr. Tenpenny is the first physician to offer documented proof that vaccines compromise the immune system.

Immunization - The Reality Behind the Myth
- Walene James
This is the only book that explores the vaccination issues from a political, ethical, psychological, aesthetic, and spiritual perspective. The author's controversial position is supported throughout the book by the scientific discoveries of researchers who have received little recognition in orthodox medical literature.

The Vaccine Book
- Dr. Robert Sears MD

An indispensable and comprehensive guide for parents facing the question – "Should I vaccinate my child?" This is an authoritative, impartial, fact-based guide to childhood vaccinations.

The Peanut Allergy Epidemic
- Heather Fraser

Essential foundational reading for parents to understand how life threatening allergies to everyday foods became epidemic. This is a vital, groundbreaking book that provides compelling evidence that allergies, as a mass phenomenon, were ushered in with the introduction and the use of vaccines and injectable medicines.

The Vaccine Friendly Plan
- Dr. Paul Thomas MD

Dr. Thomas is a vaccine-friendly Doctor knowledgeable about the latest scientific research, the community's risk for disease exposure, and a family's risk factors, health history and concerns.

Miller's Review of Critical Vaccine Studies
- Neil Z. Miller

Miller's review of critical vaccine studies contains summaries of 400 important scientific papers to help parents, governments, and researchers understand that vaccines can cause harm.

DVDs

The Greater Good

This excellent documentary increases awareness of the vaccine controversy. The film highlights personal stories of vaccine injuries and includes interviews with scientists and medical doctors on both sides of the issue.

Vaxxed: From Cover-up to Catastrophe

This documentary investigates how the CDC, the government agency charged with protecting the health of American citizens, destroyed data on a 2004 study that showed a link between the MMR vaccine and autism.

Dare to Question

The Truth About Vaccines
This comprehensive seven-part series offers an in-depth review of the history of vaccines, and a thorough analysis of the various vaccines components. This series examines safety, effectiveness and vaccine recommendations. Included are interviews with dozens of doctors, scientists, and researchers.

Online Resources

Vaccine Choice Canada – www.vaccinechoicecanada.com

Vaxxed – vaxxedthemovie.com

The Thinking Moms' Revolution - thinkingmomsrevolution.com

National Vaccine Information Centre – www.nvic.org

Learn the Risk - LearnTheRisk.org

Vaccine Truth - VacTruth.org

Age of Autism – ageofautism.com

Vaccine Resistance Movement – www.vaccineresistancemovement.org

The Weston A. Price Foundation - www.westonaprice.org/vaccinations

Product Information Inserts – http://www.vaccinesafety.edu/package_inserts.htm

Dare to Question – www.daretoquestionvaccination.com

Vaccination is exhibited on one hand as a cut and dried example
of scientists in unanimous and triumphant agreement,
while, on the other hand,
it is guarded ferociously from dissenting voices.
Discussion is actively stifled.

It is a procedure which science can neither
explain satisfactorily, nor produce robust evidence for.
In fact, believers have ruled that vaccines are not to be tested
via the rigorous randomized controlled experimental standards,
which apply to other treatments.

~ Walene James
Author – *The Vaccine Religion*

Iatrogenic (doctor caused) diseases are the third leading cause of death in the US with figures ranging from 235,000 to 284,000 deaths per year (2000).

These figures do not include deaths and injuries incurred in hospitals from unnecessary surgeries, medication errors, and incorrectly prescribed drugs.

It is also highly unlikely that any of these figures include vaccination injuries.

Only 15 percent of all medical treatments are supported by scientific evidence.

~ Walene James, Author
The Vaccine Religion

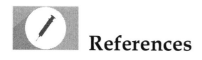 # References

Making An Informed Choice

1. **Vaccine Injury Compensation Report**
https://www.hrsa.gov/sites/default/files/hrsa/vaccine-compensation/vicp-monthly-report-12-2017.pdf

Am I The Only One

1. **Vaccine Delays, Refusals, and Patient Dismissals: A Survey of Pediatricians**
Hough-Telford K, et al. Vaccine Delays, Refusals, and Patient Dismissals: A Survey of Pediatricians. Pediatrics August 2016.

2. **L'affaire Wakefield: Shades of Dreyfus & BMJ's Descent into Tabloid Science**
http://ahrp.org/laffaire-wakefield-shades-of-dreyfus-bmjs-descent-into-tabloid-science

3. http://www.collective-evolution.com/2015/03/15/the-doctor-who-beat-the-british-general-medical-council-by-proving-that-vaccines-arent-necessary-to-achieve-health/

4. **Debate on Vaccines and Autoimmunity: Do Not Attack the Author, Yet Discuss It Methodologically.** NL Bragazzi et al. *Vaccine.* 2017 Sep 04.

18 Facts About Vaccines

1. **Canadian Immunization Schedules**
http://www.phac-aspc.gc.ca/im/ptimprog-progimpt/table-1-eng.php
http://vaccinechoicecanada.com/links/general-links/

2. **The Case For a Vaccine Injury Compensation Program for Canada**
http://www.ncbi.nlm.nih.gov/pubmed/22530534

3. **No-fault Compensation Program Overdue, Experts Say**
http://www.cmaj.ca/content/183/5/E263.full.pdf+html?sid=be18dcab-5698-481d-915c-%20c003bc404c0d

4. **Inadequate Vaccine Safety Research and Conflicts of Interest**
http://www.ebcala.org/unanswered-questions/inadequate-vaccine-safety-

Dare to Question

research-and-conflicts-of-interest

5. Hepatitis B Vaccine: Helping or Hurting Public Health?
http://www.thinktwice.com/Hep_Hear.pdf

6. Neurologic Adverse Events Following Vaccination
http://www.rescuepost.com/files/prog-health-sci-2012-vol-2-no1-neurologic-adverse-events-vaccination.pdf

7. CDC confirms the vaccine schedule and injected aluminum has never been tested   http://imgur.com/b7VfS9L

8. Combining Childhood Vaccines in One Visit Is Not Safe Journal of American Physicians and Surgeons Volume 21 Number 2 Summer 2016 http://www.jpands.org/vol21no2/miller.pdf

9. State of Health of Unvaccinated Children
http://www.vaccineinjury.info/survey/results-unvaccinated/results-illnesses.html

10. Study: Vaccinated Children Have 2 to 5 Times More Diseases and Disorders Than Unvaccinated Children
http://healthimpactnews.com/2011/new-study-vaccinated-children-have-2-to-5-times-more-diseases-and-disorders-than-unvaccinated-children

11. Thimerosal Containing Vaccines and Neurodevelopment Outcomes
http://vaccinechoicecanada.com/vaccine-ingredients/thimerosal-containing-vaccines-and-neurodevelopment-outcomes

12. Safe Minds. Research Publications 2000-2013
http://www.safeminds.org/wp-content/uploads/2013/04/SafeMinds-research-publications-2000- 2013-with-intro-FINAL.pdf

13. A two-phase study evaluating the relationship between thimerosal-containing vaccine administration and the risk for an autism spectrum disorder diagnosis in the United States
Transl Neurodegener 2013; 2 (1): 25.8. Geier DA, Hooker BS, Kern JK, et al.

14. The risk of neurodevelopmental disorders following a thimerosal-preserved DtaP formulation in comparison to its thimerosal-reduced formulation in the

Vaccine Adverse Event Reporting System (VAERS) J Biochem Pharmacol Res 2014;2(2):64-73.9. Geier DA, Kern JK, King PG, Sykes LK, Geier MR.

15. An assessment of the impact of thimerosal on childhood neurodevelopmental disorders. Pediatr Rehabil 2003; 6 (2): 97-102. Geier DA, Geier MR.

16. Aluminum, Autism and Alzheimer's
http://vaccinechoicecanada.com/in-the-news/aluminum-autism-and-alzheimers

17. Aluminum Exposure in Neonatal Patients Using the Least Contaminated Parenteral Nutrition Solution Products
http://www.ncbi.nlm.nih.gov/pmc/articles/PMC3509507

18. Aluminum, Autism and Alzheimer's
http://vaccinechoicecanada.com/in-the-news/aluminum-autism-and-alzheimers

19. Aluminum-based adjuvants should not be used as placebos in clinical trials. Vaccine, 2011 Nov 21;29(50):9289. Doi: 10.1016
http://www.ncbi.nlm.nih.gov/pubmed/21871940

20. U.S. Department of Health and Human Services. National Vaccine Injury Compensation Program. Data and Statistics.
https://www.hrsa.gov/vaccinecompensation/data/

21. Unanswered Questions from the Vaccine Injury Compensation Program: A Review of Compensated Cases of Vaccine-Induced Brain Injury
http://digitalcommons.pace.edu/pelr/vol28/iss2/6

22. A measles outbreak at a college with a prematriculation immunization requirement. Am J Public Health, 1991 Mar:81 (3):360-4.
http://www.ncbi.nlm.nih.gov/pubmed/1994745

23. DtaP and Tdap Vaccines Are Not Protective Against Whooping Cough & Are Spreading Infection
http://vaxtruth.org/2015/11/pertussis-resources

24. Immunized People Getting Whooping Cough
http://www.kpbs.org/news/2014/jun/12/immunized-people-getting-

whooping-cough

25. **What's Really Behind the Current Measles Outbreak?**
http://www.activistpost.com/2015/02/whats-really-behind-current-measles.html

26. **GlaxoSmithKline fined $3B after bribing doctors to increase drugs sales.**
https://www.theguardian.com/business/2012/jul/03/glaxosmithkline-fined-bribing-doctors- pharmaceuticals?CMP=share_btn_fb

27. **Merck: Corporate Rap Sheet**
http://www.corp-research.org/merck

28. **Brian Hooker's Findings Are Confirmed By CDC's Results**
http://www.autisminvestigated.com/brian-hooker-confirmed-by-cdc

29. **Dr. Andrew Wakefield Speaks Out on CDC Vaccine Science**
http://www.ageofautism.com/2015/08/dr-andrew-wakefield-speaks-out-on-cdc-vaccine-science.html?utm_source=feedburner&utm_medium=email&utm_campaign=Feed%3A+ageofautism +%28AGE+OF+AUTISM%29

30. **US Congressman Bill Posey (R-FL), Transcript of his speech:**
http://www.ageofautism.com/2015/07/breaking-news-congressman-posey-on-house-floor-cdc-authors-of-2004-mmr-paper-destroyed-documents.html

31. Zablotsky B, Black LI, Blumberg SJ. **Estimated prevalence of children with diagnosed developmental disabilities in the United States, 2014–2016.** *NCHS Data Brief*, no 291. Hyattsville, MD: National Center for Health Statistics. 2017

32. **Why Do Pediatricians Deny The Obvious?**
http://vaccinechoicecanada.com/health-risks/why-do-pediatricians-deny-the-obvious

33. **Chronic Illness an the State of Our Children's Health**
https://www.focusforhealth.org/chronic-illnesses-and-the-state-of-our-childrens-health/?gclid=EAIaIQobChMI6MeMkavV2AIVHlgNCh1kbQJMEAAYASAAEgJxKvD_BwE

Is The Delivery System Safe?

1. http://vaccinecommonsense.com/category/doctors/dr-todd-m-elsner/

2. **Thimerosal Containing Vaccines and Neurodevelopment Outcomes**
http://vaccinechoicecanada.com/vaccine-ingredients/thimerosal-containing-vaccines-and-neurodevelopment-outcomes

3. **Safe Minds. Research Publications 2000-2013**
http://www.safeminds.org/wp-content/uploads/2013/04/SafeMinds-research-publications-2000-2013-with-intro-FINAL.pdf

4. **A two-phase study evaluating the relationship between thimerosal-containing vaccine administration and the risk for an autism spectrum disorder diagnosis in the United States.** Transl Neurodegener 2013; 2 (1): 25.8. Geier DA, Hooker BS, Kern JK, et al.

5. **The risk of neurodevelopmental disorders following a thimerosal-preserved DtaP formulation in comparison to its thimerosal-reduced formulation in the Vaccine Adverse Event Reporting System (VAERS).** J Biochem Pharmacol Res 2014;2(2):64-73.9. Geier DA, Kern JK, King PG, Sykes LK, Geier MR.

6. **An assessment of the impact of thimerosal on childhood neurodevelopmental disorders.** Pediatr Rehabil 2003; 6 (2): 97-102. Geier DA, Geier MR.

7. **Determining the Impact of Chemical Contamination on Human Health**
https://www.cma.ca/Assets/assets-library/document/en/advocacy/PD11-11-e.pdf

8. **Vaccine Papers. An Objective Look at Vaccine Dangers.**
http://vaccinepapers.org

9. **Aluminium Exposure in Neonatal Patients Using the Least Contaminated Parenteral Nutrition Solution Products**
http://www.ncbi.nlm.nih.gov/pmc/articles/PMC3509507

10. **Study Finds Some Highest Values Aluminium Human Brain Tissue Yet-Recorded**
http://www.greenmedinfo.com/blog/study-finds-some-highest-values-aluminium-human-brain-tissue-yet-recorded-brains-

11. **Vaccine Ingredients – A Comprehensive Guide**
http://www.cdc.gov/vaccines/pubs/pinkbook/downloads/appendices/B/excipient-table-2.pdf

12. **Vaccine Ingredients**
http://vaccinechoicecanada.com/about-vaccines/vaccine-ingredients/

Dare to Question

13. **Toxicology: the Basic Science of Poisons.** Klassen C.D., editor. Casaret & Doull's, 1996

14. **Retroviruses: Poorly Understood Agents of Change**
https://www.naturalblaze.com/2017/09/retroviruses-chronic-inflammatory-disease.html

15. **Vaccines: A Reappraisal.** Richard Moskowitz, MD. Skyhorse Publishing, 2017. P. 203.

16. **Epidemiologic and Molecular Relationship Between Vaccine Manufacture and Autism Spectrum Disorder Prevalence**
https://soundchoice.s3.amazonaws.com/soundchoice/wp-content/uploads/Deisher-article-2-FINAL1.pdf

17. **Protecting Your Baby's Health.** Edda West. Vaccinechoicecanada.com

18. **The Toxins That Threaten our Brains**; The Atlantic, March 18, 2014:
https://www.theatlantic.com/health/archive/2014/03/the-toxins-that-threaten-our-brains/284466/

19. **Neonatal Immunity: The First Three Years.** Vaccine Papers & Suzanne Humphries MD video lecture.

20. **The Danger of Excessive Vaccination During Brain Development.** Russell L. Blaylock, MD. https://vaccinechoicecanada.com/wp-content/uploads/Blaylock-vaccine-autism.pdf

21. **The Immune System and Developmental Programming of Brain and Behavior.** https://www.ncbi.nlm.nih.gov/pmc/articles/PMC3484177/

22. **Vaccine Papers – An extensive look at vaccine dangers & detailed analysis of the published scientific literature**: http://vaccinepapers.org/

23. **Does an Elevated Aluminum Burden From Vaccine Adjuvants Contribute to the Rising Prevalence of Autism?** Lucija Tomljenovic, PhD & Chris Shaw, PhD. https://www.ncbi.nlm.nih.gov/pubmed/22099159

24. **Aluminum Vaccine Adjuvants: Are they Safe?** Lucija Tomljenovic, PhD & Chris Shaw, PhD. https://www.ncbi.nlm.nih.gov/pubmed/22099159

Is Vaccine Science Trustworthy?

1. **The CDC Is Being Influenced By Corporate and Political Interests.**
http://thehill.com/blogs/pundits-blog/healthcare/301432-the-cdc-is-being-being-influenced-by-corporate-and-political

2. Vaccine Papers. An Objective Look at Vaccine Dangers.
http://vaccinepapers.org

3. Let's Talk About Herd Immunity
https://leviquackenboss.wordpress.com/tag/measles/

4. A Measles Outbreak At a College With a Prematriculation Immunization
Requirement http://www.ncbi.nlm.nih.gov/pubmed/1994745

5. DtaP and Tdap Vaccines Are Not Protective Against Whooping Cough & Are
Spreading Infection http://vaxtruth.org/2015/11/pertussis-resources

6. Immunized People Getting Whooping Cough
http://www.kpbs.org/news/2014/jun/12/immunized-people-getting-whooping-cough

7. What's Really Behind the Current Measles Outbreak?
http://www.activistpost.com/2015/02/whats-really-behind-current-measles.html

8. What Would Happen If Too Many People Stopped Vaccinating?
http://immunityeducationgroup.org/happen-many-people-stopped-vaccinating/

9. An Open Letter to Legislators Currently Considering Vaccine Legislation
from Tetyana Obukhanych, PhD
http://vaccinechoicecanada.com/wp-content/uploads/Letter-to-Legislatures-Considering-Vaccine-Legislation-Obukhanych.pdf

10. Aluminium-based Adjuvants Should Not Be Used As Placebos In Clinical
Trials. Vaccine. 2011 Nov 21;29(50):9289. Doi: 10.1016
http://www.ncbi.nlm.nih.gov/pubmed/21871940

11. Vaccines: A Reappraisal. Richard Moskowitz, MD. Skyhorse Publishing, 2017.
pp. 99 – 103.

12. 144 Research Papers Supporting the Vaccine-Autism Link
https://www.scribd.com/doc/220807175/128-Research-Papers-Supporting-the-Vaccine-Autism-Link

13. http://digitalcommons.pace.edu/pelr/vol28/iss2/6

14. What the News Isn't Saying About Vaccine-Autism Studies
https://sharylattkisson.com/what-the-news-isnt-saying-about-vaccine-autism-studies

15. Vaccination: The Neurological Poison So Common Your Doctor Probably
Pushes It. Mercola.com Apr. 11, 2012.

Dare to Question

Is Measles A Manufactured Crisis?

1. **How to Repair Children Damaged By Mercury, Medicine and Politics.** Dr Michal Sichel. Fountaindale Books, 2007.

Is Vaccine Policy Sound?

1. **Universal Declaration On Bioethics and Human Rights.**
http://unesdoc.unesco.org/images/0017/001798/179844e.pdf

Is The Claim Of Vaccine Safety Valid?

1. **The List of Ingredients and Documented Side Effects**
http://healthwyze.org/reports/60-vaccine-secrets

2. **U.S. Department of Health and Human Services. National Vaccine Injury Compensation Program. Data and Statistics.**
http://www.hrsa.gov/vaccinecompensation/data/statisticsreport.pdf

3. **Pilot Comparative Study On The Health of Vaccinated and Unvaccinated 6- to 12- Year Old U.S. Children**
http://web.archive.org/web/20170504215400/http://oatext.com/Pilot-comparative-study-on-the-health-of-vaccinated-and-unvaccinated-6-to-12-year-old-U.S.-children.php

4. **Relative trends in hospitalizations and mortality among infants by the number of vaccine doses and age, based on the Vaccine Adverse Event Reporting System** (VAERS), 1990-2010. Goldman GS, Miller NZ (2012). *Hum Exp Toxicol* 31: 1012-1021.

5. **Combining Childhood Vaccines at One Visit Is Not Safe.**
   Neil Z. Miller. Journal of American Physicians and Surgeons. Summer 2016.
http://www.jpands.org/jpands2102.htm

6. **Is "Delitigation" Associated with a Change in Product Safety? The Case of Vaccines.** *Review of Industrial Organization.* July 2017.

7. **National Vaccine Information Center Vaccine Safety Science Gap Key Points**
http://www.nvic.org/PDFs/IOM/2013researchgapsIOMchildhoodimmunization schedulea.aspx

8. **CDC Confirms the Vaccine Schedule and Injected Aluminium Has Never Been Tested**
http://imgur.com/b7VfS9L

9. Vaccine Safety Science Gap Key Points Summary of 2013 IOM Report on The Childhood Immunization Schedule and Safety.

10. The Childhood Immunization Schedule and Safety: Stakeholder Concerns, Scientific Evidence, and Future Studies.
https://www.ncbi.nlm.nih.gov/books/NBK206940/

11. Vaccines: A Reappraisal. Richard Moskowitz, MD. Skyhorse Publishing, 2017. pp. 34 – 37.

12. Infant mortality rates regressed against number of vaccine doses routinely given: Is there a biochemical or synergistic toxicity? Neil Z Miller and Gary S Goldman http://journals.sagepub.com/doi/abs/10.1177/0960327111407644

13. International Comparisons of Infant Mortality
https://www.cdc.gov/nchs/data/nvsr/nvsr63/nvsr63_05.pdf

14. Infant Mortality Rates Regressed Against Number of Vaccine Doses Routinely Given: Is There a Biochemical or Synergistic Toxicity?
https://www.ncbi.nlm.nih.gov/pmc/articles/PMC3170075/

15. The Introduction of Diphtheria-Tetanus-Pertussis and Oral Polio Vaccine Among Young Infants in an Urban African Community: A Natural Experiment
http://www.ebiomedicine.com/article/S2352-3964(17)30046-4/abstract

16. https://ecf.cofc.uscourts.gov/cgi-bin/show_public_doc?2013vv0611-73-0

17. Combining Childhood Vaccines in One Visit Is Not Safe.
http://www.jpands.org/vol21no2/miller.pdf

Are Vaccines Effective?

1. The Emerging Risks of Live Virus & Virus Vectored Vaccines: Vaccine Strain, Virus Infection, Shedding & Transmission
http://www.nvic.org/CMSTemplates/NVIC/pdf/Live-Virus-Vaccines-and-Vaccine-Shedding.pdf

2. Maternally Derived Measles Immunity In Era of Vaccine-Protected Mothers.
https://www.ncbi.nlm.nih.gov/m/pubmed/3701511/

3. The Untold Story of Measles
http://business.financialpost.com/fp-comment/lawrence-solomon-the-untold-story-of-measles

4. Vaccines: A Reappraisal.
Richard Moskowitz, MD. Skyhorse Publishing, 2017. Pp. 9 – 17.

5. Seasonal Influenza Vaccine and Increased Risk of Pandemic A/H1N1-Related Illness: First Detection of the Association in British Columbia, Canada
https://academic.oup.com/cid/article/51/9/1017/292207/Seasonal-Influenza-Vaccine-and-Increased-Risk-of

6. **Association of Spontaneous Abortion With Receipt of Inactivated Influenza Vaccine Containing H1N1pdm09 in 2010–11 and 2011–12**. *Vaccine*, Volume 35, Issue 40, Pages 5314-5322

Is Vaccine History Accurate?

1. **The Smallpox Vaccine Was No Silver Bullet**
http://www.thevaccinereaction.org/2017/06/the-smallpox-vaccine-was-no-silver-bullet/

2. **Smoke And Mirrors And The Disappearance of Polio.**
http://drsuzanne.net/wp-content/uploads/2012/07/Smoke-Mirrors-and-the-%E2%80%9CDisappearance%E2%80%9D-Of-Polio-_-International-Medical-Council.pdf

3. **Dissolving Illusions: Disease, Vaccines, and The Forgotten History**. Suzanne Humphries MD, Roman Bystrianyk, 2015.

4. **Trends in Nonpolio Acute Flaccid Paralysis Incidence in India 2000 to 2013**
http://pediatrics.aappublications.org/content/135/Supplement_1/S16.2

5. **Consumer Safety Act of 1972**. Hearings before the subcommittee – United States Senate, April 20, 21 and May 3, 4, 1972. www.vaccinationcouncil.org

6. **Cancer Risk Associated With Simian Virus 40 Contaminated Polio Vaccine.**
https://www.ncbi.nlm.nih.gov/pubmed/10472327

7. **What Would Happen If Too Many People Stopped Vaccinating?**
http://immunityeducationgroup.org/happen-many-people-stopped-vaccinating/

8. **Why Do Pediatricians Deny The Obvious?**
   http://vaccinechoicecanada.com/health-risks/why-do-pediatricians-deny-the-obvious

9. **Chronic Illness an the State of Our Children's Health**
https://www.focusforhealth.org/chronic-illnesses-and-the-state-of-our-childrens-health/?gclid=EAIaIQobChMI6MeMkavV2AIVHlgNCh1kbQJMEAAYASAAEgJx KvD_BwE

10. Vaccine Injury Compensation Report
https://www.hrsa.gov/sites/default/files/hrsa/vaccine-compensation/vicp-monthly-report-12-2017.pdf

Can Vaccine Oversight Be Trusted?

1. Electronic Support for Public Health–Vaccine Adverse Event Reporting System
https://healthit.ahrq.gov/sites/default/files/docs/publication/r18hs017045-lazarus-final-report-2011.pdf

2. Vaccine Safety – CDC
https://www.cdc.gov/vaccinesafety/ensuringsafety/history/index.html

3. GlaxoSmithKline Fined $3B After Bribing Doctors to Increase Drug Sales.
https://www.theguardian.com/business/2012/jul/03/glaxosmithkline-fined-bribing-doctors-pharmaceuticals?CMP=share_btn_fb

4. Merck: Corporate Rap Sheet
http://www.corp-research.org/merck

5. Global Vaccine Market Revenues from 2014 – 2020.
https://www.statista.com/statistics/265102/revenues-in-the-global-vaccine-market/

6. Vaccine Safety Science Gap Key Points Summary of 2013 IOM Report on The Childhood Immunization Schedule and Safety.

7. Vaccines: A Reappraisal. Richard Moskowitz, MD. Skyhorse Publishing, 2017. pp. 34 – 37.

8. Vaccines: A Reappraisal. Richard Moskowitz, MD. Skyhorse Publishing, 2017. pp. 99 – 102.

If Not Vaccines, Then What?

1. New Parent Guide – Vaccine Choice Canada
https://vaccinechoicecanada.com/about-vaccines/vaccination-the-basics/parents-guide-to-vaccination/

2. The Role of Public Health Improvements in Health Advances:
The 20th Century United States
https://pdfs.semanticscholar.org/53dd/d27bc5273213c0bc7c395998911ede074833.pdf

Dare to Question

The absence of real scientific evidence of vaccine safety and effectiveness leads informed parents to conclude the vaccination paradigm is ideology rather than evidence-based medicine; and more akin to religion than science.

Parents whose children have been harmed are no longer accepting the vaccine ideology on faith. Their trust has been broken.

~ Ted Kuntz, Parent and Author
How Can I Wake Up When I Don't Know I'm Asleep?

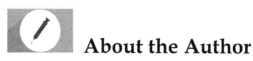

About the Author

Ted Kuntz is a father, a medical choice activist, author and educator. Kuntz's journey to examine the claims of the vaccine industry began after his son Joshua was neurologically injured by the diphtheria-pertussis-tetanus shot (DPT) in 1984.

Kuntz began a journey to understand what happened to his son. This journey revealed that the vaccine industry has been systematically and intentionally dishonest with health consumers and governments on the safety, effectiveness and necessity of vaccinations.

Kuntz believes the organized and intentional effort to deny citizens their right to make medical decisions for themselves and their children is the greatest threat to humanity today. If we lose the capacity for choice over what is injected into ourselves and our children, if we lose our self-autonomy and bodily integrity, then we are no longer free citizens.

Protecting medical choice and demanding honesty, integrity and accountability in the vaccine industry have become the most important issues in Kuntz's life.

Ted Kuntz is the author of *'Peace Begins With Me'* and *'How Can I Wake Up When I Don't Know I'm Asleep?'* Kuntz is a member of the Board of Directors of Vaccine Choice Canada and Health Action Network Society.

Kuntz's son Josh passed away in February 2017 after a life of uncontrolled seizures and diminished capacity due to vaccine induced neurological injury.

The tendency of a mass vaccination program is to herd people.
People are not cattle or sheep. They should not be herded.

~ Statement from Clinton R. Miller, Intensive Immunization
Programs, May 15th and 16th, 1962.
Hearings before the Committee on Interstate and Foreign
Commerce House of Representatives, 87th
Congress, second session on H.R. 10541.

There is evidence that the great number of vaccines
given to our children and adults,
is causing injury to their nervous systems
and that it reduces the ability of people to think, learn,
behave, and function as normal adults.

~ Dr. Russell Blaylock, MD, Neurosurgeon

Support for Dare to Question

I doubt there is a clearer, more concise, honest discourse from a parent about the vaccine industry and parents' significant vaccine concerns. The global reality that parents are facing when it comes to their most precious resources - their children's health and well-being - has, I believe, been undermined and attacked by the vaccine industry for some time now. Considering that the vaccine industry is wholly exempt from liability of any kind while constantly adding more and more vaccines to kids' schedules - with hardly any testing - is "suspicious" to say the least.

The dramatic, irrefutable statistics highlighting the current reality of the 20th and 21st centuries health epidemics in children illustrate how brain damaged and sick today's children have become - I believe, quite possibly, from vaccine products.

The startling statistics point directly into the heart of a "common denominator" link to infants and children's bizarre, sudden illnesses and brain damage through too many, too fast, injections of vaccines that contain extremely questionable ingredients for human beings. All of this is loud and clear in your book.

Superb use of John Rappoport's illustration of how an inordinate number of this century's corporate frauds can function - and thrive - by buying the media, the medical professions and government bureaucrats, while discrediting any person who "dares to question".

The Vaccine Industry, harnessing the media, smears, silences and discredits far too many experts in medical fields. Experts who have the credentials to voice their observations and knowledge about vaccines.

But the most egregious and disturbing aspect to the vaccine dilemma is the attacking and belittling of the parents' common sense concerns about their children's health. When parents have serious concerns and questions about the vaccine industry products, or about their brain damaged or dead child, the vaccine industry is twisting the parents' concerns into derogatory "anti-vaccine" propaganda.

Dare to Question

*Upon reading through again, to the last page of your book **Dare to Question**, I felt a distinct wave of peace and hope for my children who are choosing to not risk vaccinations until the industry is cleaned up and until the vaccines are proven to be safe, effective, clean, and necessary - for themselves and for their infants, toddlers and school age children.*

My adult children already know that their punishment will be ostracization, bullying, videos in the school portraying parents and children who don't vaccinate as 20th century monsters, forced home schooling, possible monetary fines and possibly jail or removal of their children - while paying taxes for schools that they will not be allowed to access. Well, so be it. At least their children will not be brain damaged for the rest of their lives by an industry that is rapidly losing credibility.

I have hope that today's parents will be heard loud and clear by the vaccine industry, and by our governments (Federal and Provincial), who should be listening to and backing the parents concerns. It is extremely disturbing that governments elected by the people, are choosing to ignore the parents concerns for their children...choosing to throw their full weight behind new legislation to support the vaccine industry.

Medical and Pediatric associations also appear to be ignoring or somehow threatening punishment for any medical professionals speaking out about the vaccine damage they are experiencing in their practices and in the emergency departments of our hospitals.

I have hope, from your well-written, concise, and honest investigations into the realities of the out of control vaccine industry, that parents will not be broken by the propaganda and vaccine bullying they are experiencing in their schools - where corporate agendas should not be by-passing parental concerns for the health and safety of their children.

We must all "Dare to Believe" that parents must be and will be the force to make the vaccine industry safe for all infants and children - parents must continue to rally, as they have already begun to take to the streets, globally, to protect their most precious of resources - their children.

Bravo! Ted Kuntz, and thank you.

Catherine Elcombe

134

Your book is simply perfect.

I feel privileged to be one of a few people who had (I won't say pleasure) an opportunity to read it. I cannot wait for its publication, because every day it goes unpublished is a waste of time. Not only is it comprehensive, but you dealt with every single aspect of this demonic panacea.

It is a great manual of common sense. You are what we consider a true intellectual. An expert on the vaccine subject and a parent of a child lost to this crime. Mine is still alive, but the quality of life spent in a residential treatment as of this June is a replica of life. I was hopeful I will eradicate/ameliorate it, but, as you have mentioned a couple of times, it is irreversible and the animal cells remain there forever.

Your book vocalizes the thoughts, sentiments, suspicions, speculations, fears of millions, except you are the one who put it so eloquently. You have also proven every single point with strong scientific and empirical arguments.

Bravo!

Again, I cannot wait for it to reach wider audiences.

Respectfully,

J. Radoman, Toronto

Dare to Question is a clear, concise inquiry, an antidote to the betrayal of science, which engages the reader to ask simple yet important questions. The Vaccine paradigm is not only broken, but one which is leading us down a path to our own demise. We must learn to dare again, and to restore what is left of our inalienable health freedom. That process of rebuilding begins with questioning our doctors, questioning the science on vaccines, and holding our heads high in these contentious times of universal deceit.

Joel Lord, founder of the Vaccine Resistance Movement

When you are studying any matter, or considering any philosophy,
ask yourself only what are the facts and what is the truth
that the facts bear out.

Never let yourself be diverted either by what you wish to believe,
or by what you think would have beneficent social effects if it were
believed.
But look only, and solely, at what are the facts.

~ Bertrand Russell

We have to lose the mystique of vaccines.
They are just products with slick sales people.

~ James Lyons-Weiler, Ph.D.

In Appreciation

This book would not have been written without the wisdom, support and efforts of many people. I would first like to express my appreciation to all those courageous researchers and scientists, politicians and parents who had the courage to tell the truth in the face of relentless resistance from the medical industry and mainstream media.

Next I would like to express my appreciation to those who were instrumental in the final content of this book. This includes Edda West, Lorna Hancock, and Joel and Margaret Sussmann, whose editorial contributions were invaluable.

Finally I would like to acknowledge the support and encouragement of my wife Darlene and my brother Tom.

And thank you to all the parents with the courage and curiousity to thoughtfully consider this information. May it serve your families well.

Ted Kuntz

For more information, and to download
a free copy of **Dare To Question** visit:

www.daretoquestionvaccination.com